Current and Future Developments in Surgery

(Volume 3)

(The Multi-Organ Donor: A-Guide to Selection, Preservation and Procurement)

Edited by

Robert S.D. Higgins & Juan A. Sanchez

Johns Hopkins University School of Medicine, Baltimore, MD, USA

Current and Future Developments in Surgery

Volume # 3

The Multi-Organ Donor: A-Guide to Selection, Preservation and Procurement

Editors: Robert S.D. Higgins & Juan A. Sanchaz

ISSN (Online): 2589-1758

ISSN (Print): 2589-174X

ISBN (Online): 978-1-68108-756-6

ISBN (Print): 978-1-68108-757-3

General:

1. Any dispute or claim arising out of or in connection with this License Agreement or the Work (including non-contractual disputes or claims) will be governed by and construed in accordance with the laws of the U.A.E. as applied in the Emirate of Dubai. Each party agrees that the courts of the Emirate of Dubai shall have exclusive jurisdiction to settle any dispute or claim arising out of or in connection with this License Agreement or the Work (including non-contractual disputes or claims).
2. Your rights under this License Agreement will automatically terminate without notice and without the need for a court order if at any point you breach any terms of this License Agreement. In no event will any delay or failure by Bentham Science Publishers in enforcing your compliance with this License Agreement constitute a waiver of any of its rights.
3. You acknowledge that you have read this License Agreement, and agree to be bound by its terms and conditions. To the extent that any other terms and conditions presented on any website of Bentham Science Publishers conflict with, or are inconsistent with, the terms and conditions set out in this License Agreement, you acknowledge that the terms and conditions set out in this License Agreement shall prevail.

Bentham Science Publishers Ltd.
Executive Suite Y - 2
PO Box 7917, Saif Zone
Sharjah, U.A.E.
Email: subscriptions@benthamscience.org

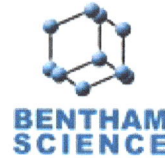

**BENTHAM
SCIENCE**

CONTENTS

PREFACE

"We make a living by what we do, but we make a life by what we give."

- *Winston Churchill*

The field of organ transplantation has evolved significantly since the first edition of this book was published in 1997. What hasn't changed is the extraordinary commitment of thousands of healthcare professionals, patients, and most importantly, donor families and loved ones who make the ultimate sacrifice in the face of a devastation loss to give the Gift of Life. These unselfish altruistic acts, which benefit dozens of potential recipients, are the cornerstones of the lifesaving benefits of organ transplantation.

Many healthcare professionals as well make significant personal and professional sacrifices to support the transplant enterprise. Without their commitment, these gifts could not be received. Over 120,000 deserving patients with end-organ failure are awaiting lifesaving or life-enhancing organ transplants. Without the commitment of the multidisciplinary teams, who in some cases have given their lives to procure these organs, the enterprise cannot succeed.

This textbook outlining the best practices in organ procurement and preservation process from world class transplant teams is dedicated to the donors and healthcare professionals who give their lives so that others could live. Special thanks to our families, including spouses, children and support staff at home, who sacrificed and supported our professional aspirations to participate in the transplant enterprise. And special thanks to Elisa Wise for her commitment to this project – which could not have come to fruition without her effort.

Robert S.D. Higgins
Johns Hopkins University School of Medicine,
Baltimore, MD
USA

List of Contributors

Ahmet Kilic	Johns Hopkins University School of Medicine, Baltimore, MD, USA
Amer Rajab	The Ohio State University, Columbus, OH, USA
Andrew Cameron	Johns Hopkins School of Medicine, Baltimore, MD, USA
Arman Kilic	University of Pittsburgh, Pittsburgh, PA, USA
Ashraf El-Hinnawi	The Ohio State University, Columbus, OH, USA
Benjamin Philosophe	Johns Hopkins University School of Medicine, Baltimore, MD, USA
Bryan Whitson	The Ohio State University, Columbus, OH, USA
Charles Alexander	The Living Legacy Foundation, Baltimore, MD, USA
Diana Greene-Chandos	The Ohio State University, Columbus, OH, USA
Dorry Segev	Johns Hopkins University School of Medicine, Baltimore, MD, USA
Eliza Beal	The Ohio State University, Columbus, OH, USA
Errol Bush	Johns Hopkins University School of Medicine, Baltimore, MD, USA
Iyore James	The Ohio State University, Columbus, OH, USA
Jaime Glorioso	Johns Hopkins University School of Medicine, Baltimore, MD, USA
Jacqueline Garonzik-Wang	Johns Hopkins University School of Medicine, Baltimore, MD, USA
Jinny Ha	Johns Hopkins University School of Medicine, Baltimore, MD, USA
Jill Buss	The Ohio State University, Columbus, OH, USA
Juan A. Sanchez	Ascension Saint Agnes Hospital, Baltimore, MD, USA
Justin Zamoyski	Fellow Neurosciences Critical Care, The Ohio State University, Columbus, OH, USA
Karen Kennedy	The Living Legacy Foundation, Baltimore, MD, USA
Kyle Jackson	Johns Hopkins School of Medicine, Baltimore, MD, USA
Marcos E. Pozo	Johns Hopkins University School of Medicine, Baltimore, MD, USA
Mitch Henry	The Ohio State University, Columbus, OH, USA
Nicole Theodoropoulos	Division of Infectious Diseases & Immunology, University of Massachusetts, Boston, MA, USA
Robert S.D. Higgins	Johns Hopkins University School of Medicine, Baltimore, MD, USA
Russell Wesson	Johns Hopkins University School of Medicine, Baltimore, MD, USA
Shane Ottmann	Johns Hopkins University School of Medicine, Baltimore, MD, USA
Sharon Weeks	Johns Hopkins University School of Medicine, Baltimore, MD, USA
Stephanie Pouch	Division of Infectious Diseases, Emory University School of Medicine, Atlanta, GA, USA
Stephen Broderick	Johns Hopkins University School of Medicine, Baltimore, MD, USA
Sylvester Black	The Ohio State University, Columbus, OH, USA

Tim Phelps   FAMI, Johns Hopkins University School of Medicine, Baltimore, MD, USA

Vincent Nardy   The Ohio State University, Columbus, OH, USA

CHAPTER 1

Introduction

Juan A. Sanchez and **Robert S.D. Higgins***

Johns Hopkins University School of Medicine, Baltimore, MD, USA

> **"Know (transplantation) and the whole of medicine is opened to you."**
>
> *-after Sir William Osler*

Keywords: Evolution of transplantation as multidisciplinary field.

The story of organ transplantation is one of remarkable achievements punctuated by spectacular breakthroughs in scientific knowledge and surgical techniques. The work of Jaboulay and Carrel in developing vascular anastomosis opened the path to the transplantation of vascularized grafts [1, 2]. The classification of histological rejection by Billingham and work by Medawar and others in immunology and cell biology created opportunities to match organs and recipients to achieve histocompatibility and to modulate the immune system and achieve tolerance as a fundamental goal for graft survival [3, 4]. The introduction of cyclosporine by Calne in 1978 heralded a new age of transplantation medicine with the development of increasingly precise agents to modulate targeted elements of the immune system and considerably extending graft survival [5]. Modern methods of preserving organs *ex vivo* have expanded the pool of organs and improve graft function. These advancements have catapulted organ transplantation from an option of the last resort to a mainline treatment for end-stage organ failure. However, although challenges continue to exist in these areas, the principal factor limiting transplantation today continues to be the shortage of suitable donor organs.

As a multidisciplinary craft, the field of transplantation touches the entire spectrum of the human experience from the most intricate cellular mechanisms, which distinguish self from foreign tissue to more abstract concepts such as altruism and societal good. It encompasses many psychological, social, economic, and regulatory aspects of human society in order to organize and maintain an

* **Corresponding author Robert S.D. Higgins:** Johns Hopkins University School of Medicine, Baltimore, MD, USA; Tel: 443-287-3497; Fax: 443-769-1273; Email: robert.higgins@jhmi.edu

equitable system of organ allocation, develop innovative outcome models, and ensuring the optimal use donor organs.

By the late 1960s, advancements in medical care and technology had improved to the point where the body could be maintained with artificial support long after the brain had irreversibly ceased to function. This required a precise definition of brain death resulting in standard set of neurologic criteria for identifying potential donors [6]. This objective determination of death was a pivotal step in organ donation which allowed retrieval of an organ in a donor before cessation of blood flow thus expanding the pool of organs beyond those which could only be recovered after the heart had stopped beating.

The Uniform Anatomical Gift Act addressing the conditions governing organ donations as well as the National Organ Transplant Act, passed by Congress in 1984, safeguarded the donation process and established a system for equitable allocation of organs to patients needing a transplant. The Social Security Act was amended in 1986 to require healthcare institutions receiving government funds to require requesting the families of potential donors about their options to donate. In 1998, federal legislation required hospitals to notify local organ procurement agencies about potential donors so that their staff could screen potential donors and offer the option of organ and tissue donation if appropriate.

Since the first publication of this book over 20 years ago, the transplant landscape has changed considerably [7]. Among the most significant of the changes is the realization that the success of transplantation is creating an ever-widening gap between demand and supply of donor organs. This has prompted the exploration of other ways to increase the pool of donors such as living organ donation, donation after circulatory death, *ex vivo* organ circulatory support, partial organ transplants, and mechanical/artificial organs. In addition, there is increasing consideration of organs from donors not previously viewed as suitable due to age and other factors (*i.e.* Hepatitis C and HIV). As such, selecting and managing potential donors are more important than ever in addition to the need to individualize, allograft selection based on the specific risk profiles of both donor and recipient in order to maximize the equitable allocation of organs and the recipient's chances for a successful outcome.

CONSENT FOR PUBLICATION

Not applicable.

CONFLICT OF INTEREST

The author declares no conflict of interest, financial or otherwise.

ACKNOWLEDGEMENTS

Declared none.

REFERENCES

[1]   Jaboulay M. Greffe du reins au pli du conde par soudures arterielles et veineuses (Kidney grafts in the antecubital fossa by arterial and venous anastomosis). Lyon Med 1906; 107: 575.

[2]   Carrel A. Results of the transplantation of blood vessels, organs and limbs. JAMA 1908; 51: 1662-7.
[http://dx.doi.org/10.1001/jama.1908.25410200010001b] [PMID: 6345837]

[3]   Billingham RE, Brent L, Medawar PB. Actively acquired tolerance of foreign cells. Nature 1953; 172(4379): 603-6.
[http://dx.doi.org/10.1038/172603a0] [PMID: 13099277]

[4]   Medawar PB. A second study of the behaviour and fate of skin homografts in rabbits. J Anat 1945; 79: 157-76.

[5]   Calne RY, White DJ, Thiru S, *et al.* Cyclosporin A in patients receiving renal allografts from cadaver donors. Lancet. 1978 Dec 23-30; 2(8104-5): 1323-7.

[6]   A definition of irreversible coma. Report of the Ad Hoc Committee of the Harvard Medical School to Examine the Definition of Brain Death. JAMA 1968; 205(6): 337-40.
[http://dx.doi.org/10.1001/jama.1968.03140320031009] [PMID: 5694976]

[7]   Higgins RSD, Sanchez JA, Baldwin JC. The Multiorgan Donor: Selection and Management. 1997; ISBN-13: pp. 978-0865423954.

CHAPTER 2

The Organ Allocation System

Karen Kennedy[*] and **Charles Alexander**

The Living Legacy Foundation, Baltimore, MD, USA

Abstract: The following chapters give a succinct reference about how the system is set up, including how organs are listed and allocated and then distributed, for a reader like a resident or fellow trying to understand how organs go from donor to implanted organs, as well as the role of the OPO and what governs your efforts and success.

Keywords: Organ Allocation, OPO, Organ Distribution.

INTRODUCTION

Organ Procurement Organizations (OPOs) serve an essential role in the coordination of organ donation processes, in partnership with transplant centers and acute care hospitals throughout the United States. Each entity has regulatory, legislative and accreditation requirements, which provide oversight to their respective functions and ensure the utmost safety for potential recipients awaiting solid organ transplants. To best outline these vital roles, a brief review of the legislative and regulatory history of organ donation and transplantation is of value.

Legislative, Regulatory and Accreditation History Highlights

As medical science advanced and solid organ transplantation increasingly became a feasible option for patients in the mid-twentieth century, the need to establish systematic processes for recipient listing and organ allocation became evident to medical professionals and legislators. In 1984, the U.S. Congress enacted the National Organ Transplant Act (NOTA) [1] to address these needs. In 1986, the Federal Omnibus Budget Reconciliation Act was enacted and included language related to developing relevant organ donation and transplantation systems [1]. Highlights of these acts include:

---

[*] **Corresponding author Karen Kennedy:** The Living Legacy Foundation, Baltimore, MD, USA; Tel: 443-414-2123; Emails: kkennedy@thellf.org; karenliangkennedy@yahoo.com

Robert S.D. Higgins & Juan A. Sanchez (Eds.)

- Establishment of the Organ Procurement and Transplantation Network (OPTN), through the Health and Human Resources Administration (HRSA), to maintain a national registry for potential recipient listing organ allocation, administered by a non-profit organization under federal contract [1]
- Creation of the Scientific Registry of Transplant Recipients (SRTR) [1], also administered through HRSA, to provide statistical and analytic support to the OPTN to help in the formulation and evaluation of organ allocation and other OPTN policies [1]
- Prohibition on the buying or selling of human organs for transplantation [1]
- OPO responsibilities in promoting organ donation, identifying potential donors, and recovering and distributing the recovered organs for transplantation [1]
- Requirements for acute care hospitals to have a working agreement with an OPO [1]

As outlined, the NOTA provisions included a mandate for the creation of an Organ Procurement and Transplantation Network (OPTN), facilitated under federal contract through HRSA. The United Network for Organ Sharing (UNOS), based in Richmond, Virginia, was awarded the first contract by the U.S. Department of Health and Human Services in 1986 [2] and has held the contract to this date. Highlights of the services provided by UNOS, as the OPTN contractor, include oversight of: the organ sharing system, equitable and timely allocation of donor organs, and promulgation of donation and transplantation related policies [2].

In collaboration with transplant centers, acute care hospitals, and HLA laboratories throughout the United States, OPOs function as an integral partner in the national organ donation and allocation systems. Their responsibilities are extensively outlined in OPTN/UNOS policies [2]; of particular importance is the scope of clinical activities they facilitate to ensure the safety of organs allocated and, as importantly, to honor the gift of organs provided by donors and their families.

The Centers for Medicaid and Medicare Services (CMS), in its Code of Federal Regulations (CFR), also have oversight of transplant centers, acute care hospitals and OPOs, as outlined in its Conditions of Participation [3]. Highlights include requirements for hospitals to implement protocols with OPOs for timely notification of every individual whose death is imminent or who has died. Extensive OPO performance and outcome metrics are also outlined, monitored and evaluated by CMS. Additionally, these requirements stipulate that OPOs maintain an advisory board with representation that includes, but is not limited to: hospital administrators, intensive care or emergency room personnel, tissue banks, voluntary health associations, histocompatibility experts, neurosurgeons or physicians with neurosciences skills, transplant surgeons from transplant center in OPO's service area, and donor family members.

CMS also designates, for each OPO, a defined geographic area or "donation service area" (DSA) [3]. OPOs are required by law to have written agreements with each hospital in its DSA, outlining its processes for organ donation, recovery and transplantation. Fig. (**2.1**) [4] outlines the current CMS defined geographic DSAs.

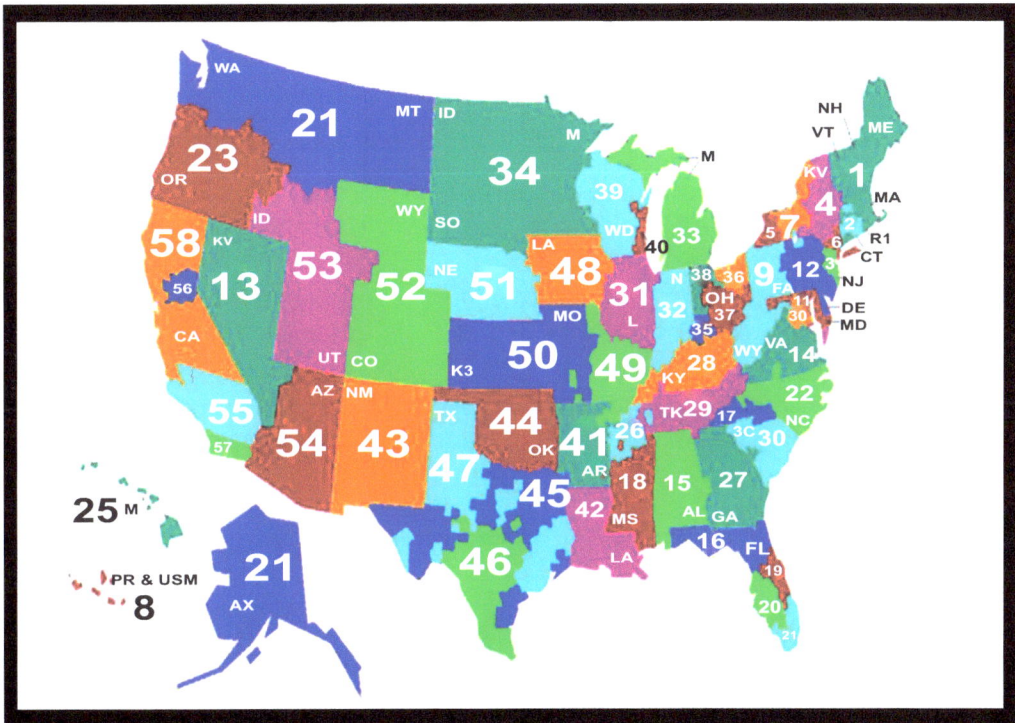

Fig. (2.1). Service areas of U.S. organ procurement organizations [4] [from Herdman & Potts, Non-Hear--Beating Organ Donation, 1997, Appendix C]. Medical Illustrations© 2018 Tim Phelps, MS, FAMI, Johns Hopkins University.

Uniform Anatomical Gift Act

The Uniform Law Commission (ULC) is a national entity that drafts model legislation for adoption into state laws on subjects for which nationwide uniformity is desirable [5]. The original 1968 Uniform Anatomical Gift Act (UAGA) was promulgated by the ULC to address the emerging regulations and laws being established related to organ and tissue donation across the United States. The original version of this Act was passed and adopted in all 50 states.

In 2006, the scope of the UAGA was revised to reflect changes across the United States related to key aspects of the donation process, to include the order for hierarchy of next of kin and the adoption of electronic signatures. Importantly, the 2006 revised UAGA [5] also strengthened prior language barring others from attempting to override an individual's decision to make or refuse to make an anatomical gift. Most states passed this legislation, with revisions as indicated, in their respective legislatures.

Among the important highlights of this model legislation [5] are provisions to:

• Honor the autonomous decision of individuals who designate their wish to be a donor through a document of gift
• Establish the hierarchy for classes of individuals who can give authorization for donation
• Outline standards that enable donor programs to gain access to documents of gift in donor registries, medical records, and records of the state motor vehicle department
• Define the circumstances in which a document of gift can be revoked
• Define the roles and responsibilities of hospitals in facilitating the referral and donation processes
• Establish the responsibilities of hospital providers in giving adequate time to donor programs to evaluate the potential suitability of donors, as well as access to any available medical records

Organ Procurement Organization Accreditation Program

The Association of Organ Procurement Organizations (AOPO) is the national non-profit organization representing the current fifty-eight federally designated OPOs [6]. In 1986, standards established by its predecessor were adopted by the Health Care Financing Administration (HCFA) when they instituted a certification process for OPOs [3]. Highlights of AOPO services include: disseminating standards for organ procurement programs, serving as the national accrediting body for OPOs, and facilitating education and research initiatives in collaboration with other healthcare organizations and federal agencies [6].

The accreditation program established by AOPO is integral to maintaining the highest standards of excellence in procurement processes and adherence to all federal laws and regulations. Accreditation, if granted, is provided after a detailed on-site survey and extensive desk audit performed by OPO practice experts. The OPO, if approved, receives accreditation for a three year period [5]; re-accreditation is subsequently required every three years.

Organ Donor Clinical Processes

The preceding historical overview provides a framework for exploring the donation and allocation process in more detail. The responsibilities of an OPO, as outlined by the regulatory and accrediting bodies, are extensive and comprehensive; they extend from the initial hospital referral to follow-up activities once the surgical recovery is complete. Their goal is to ensure organ function is maximized, all suitable organs are transplanted, and safety standards are maintained. The following sections explore specific clinical steps in the process, as illustrated in Fig. (**2.2**) (7); each OPO and transplant center operationalizes clinical practices in a manner that best meets their program's needs.

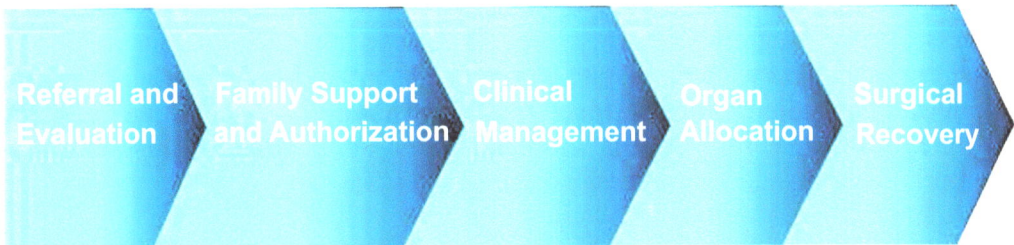

Fig. (2.2). The Living Legacy Foundation of Maryland clinical process outline [7] [From The LLF training program materials in effect April, 2018]. Medical Illustrations© 2018 Tim Phelps, MS, FAMI, Johns Hopkins University.

Referral and Evaluation

In accordance with CMS requirements, every acute care hospital has policies in place which guide staff in making potential donor referrals in a timely manner to their designated OPO [3]. Although policies vary across the United States, each program has triggers, or indicators, for when referrals should be made. The following represents an example of these triggers, as outlined in The Living Legacy Foundation OPO's Standard Operating Procedures [8]:

- Imminent deaths, as defined by the OPO and acute care hospital
- Patients with a grave neurological insult, indicated by a Glasgow Coma Score (GCS) of 3-5
- Patients who have sustained death by cardiac criteria
- Prior to the terminal extubation of a patient
- Situations in which the family initiates the topic of donation

When donation is a possibility based on the preliminary information provided, the OPO then performs a more comprehensive suitability evaluation. This evaluation is based on an extensive review of available hospital records and assessment of the current clinical treatment plan for the patient. Once initial suitability is determined, the OPO will continue to follow the patient's clinical course. When evaluating donation potential, there are many considerations [2, 7, 8], to include: age, medical history, neurological status, clinical course and potential for progression to brain death. These factors also assist in determining if a patient meets established criteria for the organ donation after cardiac death (DCD) pathway and/or the organ donation after neurological death pathway.

Authorization Processes

For a patient who meets suitability requirements, the timing for offering the opportunity for donation is determined in a collaborative manner between the healthcare and OPO teams. All families are treated with the utmost respect and sensitivity [7, 8], and ongoing support is offered by the teams throughout the process. Many programs utilize a process known as a huddle, in which the healthcare and OPO teams facilitate a brief and focused discussion (huddle) prior to offering donation options, designed to: discuss family dynamics, determine the legal next of kin, identify if a patient had made a donor designation, and assess appropriate timing and venue for the discussion [7, 8].

Each OPO operationalizes its authorization processes in a manner that meets their unique program needs and is in adherence with all regulatory and accrediting entity requirements. This process includes documentation of the authorization process completed with the next of kin, outlining the organs which have been authorized for transplant, research, education and/or medical therapy. In circumstances where an individual has designated their intent to be a donor through a document of gift as outlined in the UAGA [5], commonly known as first person authorization, the OPO will likewise work closely with the decedent's next of kin to honor their designation. OPO family services representatives also conduct a comprehensive donor risk assessment interview (DRAI) with the next of kin and any other individuals who may contribute vital information about the donor's medical and social history [2, 3, 6, 8].

Clinical Donor Management

The donor management process is complex and multi-faceted, encompassing astute assessments and targeted interventions over a broad range of parameters. OPTN/UNOS policies, AOPO standards, OPO practices and transplant center guidelines [2, 3, 6] provide the framework for the clinical management of donors. Each OPO develops clinical management processes to ensure the safety of every organ for waiting recipients. OPTN/UNOS policies offer very detailed outlines for donor related clinical responsibilities; Table **2.1** highlights OPTN/UNOS Policy 2 [2] and shows examples of the diverse scope of OPO related requirements:

Table 2.1. Excerpts from OPTN/UNOS policies related to OPO responsibilities [2] [From OPTN/UNOS policies in effect April, 2018].

Highlights of OPTN/UNOS Policy 2: Deceased Donor Organ Procurement [2]
Identify potential donors and perform suitability evaluations
Provide evidence of authorization and verify death pronounced according to applicable law
Obtain detailed donor medical and social history
Facilitate clinical management and coordinate ABO, HLA and infectious disease testing
Execute match runs to guide organ allocation
Participate in surgical recovery of organs
Coordinate labeling, packaging and transportation of organs
Ensure adequate documentation of all activities

AOPO standards and OPTN/UNOS policies [2, 6] outline specific clinical information which must be obtained to evaluate organ function for every donor; in addition, there are specific parameters for a number of organ systems. Often, additional testing or diagnostics may be indicated or requested by the OPO medical director or transplant program. Table **2.2** [2] provides examples of both required and requested information, both through UNOS and at the program's discretion. This list is not intended to be all encompassing; more detailed information can be found in individual OPO clinical management policy statements [8].

Table 2.2. Excerpts from OPTN/UNOS policies related to organ donor evaluation parameters [2] [From OPTN/UNOS policies in effect April, 2018].

Highlights of OPTN/UNOS Policy 2: Donor Evaluation Parameters [2]		
All Donors	Age, ethnicity, height, weight Clinical course, medical/social history Physical assessment ABO and subtyping, if indicated Infectious disease testing HLA typing	Blood, urine and sputum cultures Electrolytes, CBC with diff Hemodynamics Intake and output Medications and vasopressor agents Chest x-ray
Kidney	Final urinalysis, biopsies (if indicated based on donor characteristics)	
Pancreas	Serum amylase and serum lipase	

(Table 2.2) cont.....

Liver	Aspartate aminotransferase (AST) Alanine aminotransferase (ALT) Alkaline phosphatase Total and direct bilirubin	International normalized ration (INR) or Prothrombin (PT) if not available Partial thromboplastin time (PTT) Biopsy pre-operatively, if indicated based on donor characteristics
Lungs	Arterial blood gases O2 challenge Sputum gram stain Mycology sputum smear	Serial chest x-rays Bronchoscopy (if available) 12-lead electrocardiogram, echocardiogram (if OPO has facilities) Select chest measurements
Heart	Cardiac enzymes, including creatinine phosphokinase (CPK) isoenzymes 12-lead electrocardiogram Central venous pressure (CVP) or Swan Ganz instrumentation	Cardiology consult or echocardiogram (if available) Cardiac catheterization may be requested, based on donor characteristics
VCA	Specific parameters are determined by the potential recipient's needs and evaluated on a case by case basis May include additional imaging, measurements, and additional lab work	
Notes: Additional diagnostics may be requested for any organ system, based on donor's clinical presentation and could include: ultrasound, CT scan, MRI, X-rays, and additional lab work [2]		

Donor Management Priorities

The donor management phase exemplifies the collaborative nature of OPO, donor hospital and transplant center relationships in maximizing the viability of authorized organs. Clinical goals and objectives are established to optimize organ function, based on OPO policies. Key responsibilities during this phase include performing extensive organ function testing, obtaining all required lab work, and facilitating any indicated diagnostics [2, 6, 8]. Each organ donor case is unique and the OPO team, in consultation with their Medical Director, implements interventions tailored to the donor's specific clinical needs. Table **2.3** [7] represents an excerpt from an OPO donor management goals worksheet [7]:

Documentation is an essential aspect of the donation process and OPOs utilize clinical databases to record all relevant donor information. This information is ultimately provided to UNOS, which administers the computerized system known as UNet [2]. Through this system, UNOS maintains the list of potential organ recipients and serves as the repository for all organ donor data. With this data, UNOS is able to safely match those recipients with donors in the most equitable manner possible. The next section will explore the organ allocation process in more detail.

Table 2.3. Excerpt from The Living Legacy Foundation donor management guidelines [7] [From The LLF training program materials in effect April, 2018].

The Living Legacy Foundation of Maryland
Critical Care Donor Management Guidelines

GOAL: ADEQUATE OXYGENATION
$SaO_2 > 95\%$, $PaO_2 > 100mmHg$

Recommended Management:
1. Continue pulmonary hygiene measures: frequent suctioning, CPT q 4 hours, turn q 2 hours
2. Monitor trends in ABG's
3. Perform O2 challenges, per The LLF protocol
4. Add at least 5cm of PEEP for all donors; TV 8-10 cc/kg
5. Evaluate vent mode - consider PCV and APRV - done collaboratively with Medical Director
6. Updated CXR required; may need serial CXRs for lung donors
7. Reverse Trendelenburg positioning to assist with recruitment

GOAL: ADEQUATE HYDRATION AND PERFUSION
SBP 90-120 mmHg, MAP >60mmHg, CVP 5-12mmHg, Hct > 25%

Recommended Management:
1. Monitor BP, HR, Temp, and CVP, at least Q1 hour
2. Maintain volume with appropriate infusions; determined in collaboration with The LLF
3. Support BP with inotropic agents tailored to donor's specific hemodynamic needs
4. Initiate T 4 protocol - bolus and continuous infusion, titrated by The LLF coordinator
5. Blood products, FFP, platelets, cryoprecipitate may be required, as indicated

Organ Allocation Overview

All solid organs are allocated utilizing OPTN/UNOS policy [2] derived algorithms for each organ system. Specific donor and waiting recipient criterion are programmed into UNet, from which match runs are generated. A match run is a process that filters and ranks waiting list candidates based on this criteria, as well as their medical compatibility with the donor [2]. The candidate list is dynamic, based on factors such as: ABO, time waiting, geographic location, age, and medical urgency.

Each OPO has developed systems by which communication with DSA based and external transplant centers occurs when allocating organs from the match runs. Organ offers are made in a systematic process, following the sequence of candidates on the match run. Specific OPTN derived codes are utilized to document in UNet the acceptance or decline of an organ by the transplant center

[2]. This system ensures fairness and equity, by demonstrating OPO and transplant center adherence to following the exact sequence order of potential recipients on the match run.

The following discussion provides a very general overview, by organ system, of adult potential recipient listing criteria and allocation algorithms. For a more extensive review, and for specific details related to pediatric allocation, OPTN/UNOS policies serve as the definitive source [2]. It should also be noted that OPTN/UNOS policies are subject to revisions, as indicated, so referencing the OPTN website ensures access to the most current policy language [2].

Heart and Lung Wait Lists and Allocation: Excerpts from UNOS Policies 6, 10 [2]

The algorithm used to generate heart and lung match run lists are impacted in large measure by these key factors: donor and waiting recipient ABO, height, and weight; geographic location of the potential recipient relative to the donor hospital location; medical urgency; and waiting time. There are also specific considerations given to pediatric patients, depending on the acuity and severity of their illness.

With respect to heart allocation, the match run lists potential recipients based on established algorithms. Allocation for adult donors 18 years of age or older includes numerous classifications, beginning with the following (the full classifications list for adult and pediatric donors can be found in UNOS policies [2]:

- Classification 1: Candidates in the OPO's DSA or Zone A (up to 500 miles from the donor hospital) who are adult status 1 or pediatric status 1A and primary blood type match with the donor.
- Classification 2: Candidates in the OPO's DSA or Zone A (up to 500 miles from the donor hospital) who are adult status 1 or pediatric status 1A and secondary blood type match with the donor.
- Classification 3: Candidates in the OPO's DSA or Zone A (up to 500 miles from the donor hospital) who are adult status 2 and primary blood type match with the donor.

All candidates are given a status, which indicates their medical urgency and determines their waitlist sequence, as follows [2]:

- Adult Status 1A (patients ≥ 18): In transplant hospital, and has at least one of the following:
- Mechanical circulatory support *via* artificial heart, intra-aortic balloon pump, or ECMO device

- Continuous mechanical ventilation
- Continuous infusion of single high-dose or multiple intravenous inotropes (blood pressure agents)

OR

- May or may not be in transplant hospital, and has at least one of the following: VAD (ventricular assist device) or mechanical support with significant complications
- Adult Status 1B (patients ≥ 18); Patient has at least one of the following:
- VAD (ventricular assist device) or continuous infusion of intravenous inotropes
- Adult Status 2 (patients ≥ 18): Patient who does not meet criteria for 1A or 1B but suitable for transplant

With respect to lung allocation, the following considerations are integral to the process [2]:

- For potential recipients ages 12 and above, select medical information is gathered to calculate a lung allocation score (LAS), which stratifies the severity of illness on a scale from 0 to 100
- All candidates are placed in order for compatible lung offers, according to their score, within a 250 nautical mile circle around the donor hospital, and then in broader geographic zones, in a similar fashion to the heart allocation algorithm
- Pediatric recipients < 12 years of age are assigned priority for allocation based on medical urgency

Liver Wait List and Allocation: Excerpts from UNOS Policy 9 [2]

With respect to liver allocation the match run lists potential recipients according to established algorithms. Allocation for adult donors 18 years of age or older also includes numerous classifications, beginning with the following (the full classifications list for adult and pediatric donors, as well as any regional variations, can be found in UNOS policies [2]:

- Classification 1: Candidates in the OPO's region who are adult or pediatric status 1A
- Classification 2: Candidates in the OPO's region who are pediatric status 1B

Each waiting recipient is assigned a MELD (Model for End-Stage Liver Disease) or PELD (Pediatric End-Stage Liver Disease) score. This score is derived based on lab levels and other clinical factors. Liver candidates at least 18 years old at the time of registration may be assigned any of the following: Adult status 1A, Calculated MELD score, Exception MELD score or Inactive status [2]. Highlights of these priorities include [2]:

- **Adult Status 1A (patients ≥ 18):** Patient has at least one of following, with life expectancy < 7 days [2]:
- Fulminant liver failure or anhepatic state
- Primary non-function of a transplanted liver within 7 days
- Hepatic artery thrombosis in a transplanted liver within 7 days
- Acute decompensated Wilson's disease

Intestine Allocation Algorithm: Excerpts from UNOS Policy 7 [2]

The algorithm used to generate a match run for an intestine is based on these key factors: donor and recipient ABO; recipient's waiting time; medical urgency; and geographic location of recipient relative to donor hospital [2].

Geographic Location [2]

For intestine allocation, geographic location of recipients is always prioritized in this order [2]:

- Local transplant centers
- The OPO's OPTN/UNOS region
- Nationally, to other regions

Medical Urgency [2]

All candidates on the intestine waitlist are given a status that indicates their medical urgency.

Status 1: candidates with any of the following conditions [2]:

- Liver function test abnormalities
- Restriction of intravenous feeding due to absence of vascular access
- Urgent medical indications for an intestinal organ transplant

Status 2: Any candidate that does not meet requirements for Status 1

Additional Considerations

Potential recipients may be listed for the intestine alone or for multiple organs, such as liver, stomach, and/or pancreas. It is important to note that candidates for combined liver-intestine transplants must be matched by using the liver match run [2].

Kidney Wait List and Allocation: Excerpts from UNOS Policy 8 [2]

The kidney algorithm is known as the Kidney Allocation System (KAS). This algorithm is designed to make more kidneys available for transplant and increase the years of life gained per transplanted kidney. The UNOS algorithm [2] weighs the following factors:

- Donor and recipient blood type
- Donor's Kidney Donor Profile Index (KDPI) score
- Recipient's Expected Post Transplant Survival (EPTS) score
- Recipient's Calculated Panel Reactive Antibody (CPRA) percentage
- Recipient's Kidney Allocation Points score
- Antigen mismatch between the donor and recipient
- Geographic proximity of the donor and recipient

KDPI Score [2]

Each kidney offered for transplant is given a KDPI score from 0% to 100%, representing the kidney's projected longevity in comparison to other kidneys. This percentage is calculated based on the Kidney Donor Risk Index (KDRI) score [2], which considers: donor age; height; weight; ethnicity; serum creatinine level; Hepatitis C status; whether cause of death is a stroke; type of donor; and past medical history of diabetes or hypertension.

Based on this scoring system, kidneys in the upper range of function have lower KDPI percentages [2]. For example: A KDPI of 35% indicates that out of 100 kidneys, the kidney being allocated is expected to function for a longer period of time than the other 65 kidneys.

EPTS Score [2]

An EPTS score is assigned to all candidates 18 years of age and older. It incorporates four measurements: time candidate's age, dialysis status, current diabetes diagnosis and history of previously organ transplants. The score indicates the patient's expected survival time after transplant. A lower score represents an expected longer survival time. Candidates with longer than expected survival times generally are matched to kidneys that are expected to function longer and which have lower KDPI scores [2].

CPRA Percentage [2]

The candidate's CPRA percentage represents the number of HLA antibody reactions they have when their serum is tested against white blood cells from a panel of approximately 100 area blood donors. The lower the CPRA, the less reaction the candidate's blood has to samples from the panel [2]. A CPRA of 0, for example, represents zero reactions and 0% chance of acute rejection from this group of donors. A CPRA of 75, on the other hand, represents reactions to 75 out of 100 samples. Acute rejection of an organ from these donors would thus be expected to be experienced at a 75% rate [2].

KAS System [2]

The KAS system gives additional stratified points for all candidates with a CPRA levels of 20 and higher, as a higher CPRA means the candidate has a rarer chance of being matched with a compatible donor, and thus would be likely to spend more time on the waitlist [2].

Kidney Allocation Points Score [2]

In addition to receiving Kidney Allocation Points for higher CPRA scores, candidates are also given points for aspects such as lower antigen mismatches or for pediatric candidates with zero mismatch. Kidney Allocation Points more notably accrue for time spent on the waiting list; these points are used to rank candidates within the different algorithm groups [2].

Antigen Mismatch [2]

Although HLA antigen mismatch is used to calculate CPRA and to allot Kidney Allocation Points, of the six basic tissue typing antigens, HLA-A, HLA-B, and HLA-DR are also looked at directly as the antigens most influential in predicting graft survival or rejection [2]. If the transplant candidate has no direct antibodies to the donor for these antigens, the match carries a low rate of rejection and is referred to as either a 0 AB-DR mismatch or a zero antigen mismatch.

Geographic Proximity

In general, kidney allocation is geographically prioritized as follows: Local transplant centers, the OPO's OPTN/UNOS region, and then nationally to other regions [2]. It is important to note that the specific geographic sequencing varies, depending on the KDPI score [2]. and the age of the potential recipient. As with liver allocation, these differences help to prioritize pediatric patients and patients with more urgent medical need.

Double Kidney Allocation [2]

An additional consideration regarding kidney allocation relates to donors with certain specific characteristics. For a donor who meets at least two of the following criteria, both kidneys may (not required) be allocated to one recipient, at the accepting surgeon's discretion [2]:

- 60 years of age
- Estimated creatinine clearance < 65 ml/min based upon admission serum creatinine
- Rising serum creatinine (greater than 2.5 mg/dL) at time of organ recovery
- History of longstanding hypertension or diabetes mellitus
- Glomerulosclerosis >15% and < 50%

Pancreas Wait List and Allocation: Excerpts from UNOS Policy 11 [2]

If a pancreas is available for transplant, the match run list is executed as both a pancreas and kidney-pancreas waitlist. This ensure that candidates in need of both organs have equitable access to receive them when both are available [2]. It should be noted, however, that if only a pancreas is available for transplant, the OPO can offer it only to candidates who do not also need a kidney.

The algorithm used to generate the combined pancreas and kidney-pancreas match run list involves many factors, to include: CPRA percentage; antigen mismatch; geographic proximity; and waiting time [2].

CPRA Percentage [2]

As with kidney allocation, CPRA is used to indicate the HLA antibody reactions present when a candidate's serum is tested against that of approximately100 area blood donors. Again, the lower the CPRA, the less reaction the candidate is likely to manifest to samples from the panel and the lower the acute rejection rate; the higher the CPRA, the more reactions they are likely to manifest [2]. Higher CPRAs with zero mismatch are prioritized in the algorithm because these candidates would otherwise spend a longer time on the transplant list while waiting for a matching donor [2].

Antigen Mismatch [2]

As is the case for kidney allocation, HLA-A, HLA-B, and HLA-DR are examined to determine survival of the transplanted organ(s) [2]. Candidates with zero or low antibodies to the donor for these antigens are prioritized, as these matches indicate a lower rate of rejection.

Geographic Proximity and Waiting Time

In general, the geographic order for pancreas allocation is listed below; as with other organs, this is impacted by other factors, to ensure the pancreas is offered to higher priority candidates with the least chance of rejection. Within each of these categories, candidates also are sequenced based on waiting time [2]:

- Local transplant centers
- The OPO's OPTN/UNOS region
- Nationally, to other regions

Kidney - Pancreas Allocation: Excerpts from UNOS Policy 11 [2]

It is notable that if both a kidney and pancreas are available for transplant, the kidney can only be offered to candidates who are prioritized *via* the KP list, and not to candidates who appear because of their pancreas listing. There are additional factors regarding how a pancreas can be allocated when both a kidney and pancreas are available. When allocating a kidney and pancreas together, once an offer has been made to candidates in the first five categories on the match run list, the OPO can decide whether to offer the kidney and pancreas separately to candidates on the pancreas only list and kidney only list, or to keep offering to candidates on the combined list [2].

ABO

Blood type differences between pancreas-only allocation and kidney-pancreas allocation are included in the algorithm. For donors with blood types B and AB, a kidney-pancreas offer must be made to candidates with those specific blood types. For donors with blood type A, a kidney-pancreas can be offered to candidates with either A or AB blood type [2]. For donors with blood type O, a kidney-pancreas can be offered to candidates with blood type O, or any other blood type only if there is a zero antigen mismatch and a CPRA of 80% or higher [2].

VCA Wait List and Allocation: Excerpts from UNOS Policy 12 [2]

The potential recipient listing and allocation processes for vascularized composite allografts (VCA), such as face and hand transplants, were adopted in 2014. In general, the host OPO will offer VCA grafts to candidates on the waiting list with compatible blood type who are willing to accept a VCA graft with similar physical characteristics to the donor [2]. The OPO offers VCA grafts to candidates in the following order [2]: candidates within the OPO's region and then candidates beyond the OPO's region. Within these two classification, candidates are sorted by waiting time (longest to shortest).

Surgical Recovery Processes

As described by Rudow, Ohler, and Shafer [9], planning for the surgical recovery begins early in the donation process. While the OPO team is facilitating the clinical processes for organ evaluation and allocation in the donor hospital ICU or

OPO based clinical setting, they are also in close communication with the Operating Room team to establish the optimal timing for the surgical recovery [2, 8, 9].

As all suitable organs are being allocated, plans are finalized for the timing and location of the surgical recovery, which can occur at the donor hospital, or facilitated at an OPO based recovery suite. The OPO coordinates all aspects of the surgical recovery in collaboration with the donor hospital and transplant centers who have accepted organs on behalf of waiting recipients, utilizing their specific policies, and in adherence with all national regulatory and accrediting body requirements [2, 6].

The timing of the recovery is determined based on many factors, to include:

• Donor hemodynamic stability
• Donor family considerations
• Potential recipient instability
• OR availability (some OPOs have surgical suites at their facility)
• OPO or transplant center level of activities, such as multiple donor cases and/or transplants

There are numerous details addressed by the OPO during final preparations prior to the recovery. Communication with the OR team to review case priorities and equipment and supply needs are facilitated by the OPO coordinator [2, 6, 8, 9]. The on-site team also draws UNOS required specimens [2] and ensures all relevant documentation has been completed, to include: ABO confirmation, authorization and DRAI, brain death notes and/or death certificate, infectious disease results, donor clinical data, and any other information requested by the transplant surgeons [2].

An essential element of OR preparation includes verification of the credentials of all transplant center surgical recovery personnel. Per CMS regulations and AOPO standards, OPOs must have credentialing records for physicians, surgeons and other practitioners who routinely recover organs in hospitals with the OPO [2, 6, 8, 9]. OPOs address, in their respective operational policies, the scope of credentialing elements required for these recovery personnel. Additionally, for surgeons or other qualified practitioners who do not routinely recover organs on behalf of the OPO, protocols must be in place that facilitate the expeditious verification of their credentialing prior to a recovery [2, 6, 8, 9].

This process is facilitated using the AOPO Confirmation Information Network (ACIN) system [6]. All OPOs must enter specific information about the eligibility of recovery personnel in their DSA into the ACIN system. As part of the preparations for a surgical recovery, the ACIN system is accessed by the OPO staff to check the credentials for any recovery personnel participating in the recovery.

The OPO team has numerous responsibilities immediately prior to, during, and after the surgical recovery; these are all designed to ensure the safety and *via* bility of the organs provided for transplant. Table **2.4** [2] highlights these responsibilities:

Table 2.4. Excerpts from OPTN/UNOS policies related to surgical recovery priorities [2] [From OPTN/UNOS policies in effect April, 2018].

Highlights of OPTN/UNOS Policy 2: Surgical Recovery Priorities [2]	
OR Set up	Collaborate with OR staff for surgical suite set up and supply needs Set up back table for each organ Select appropriate cannulas, flush solutions and sufficient sterile topical ice Ensure any needed equipment, such as bronchoscopy cart, is available
Clinical Priorities	Collaborate with anesthesia and surgeons to monitor donor stability and implement any needed interventions Advocate for lab work or additional testing needs identified during case Ensure donor related medications, such as heparin, administered at appropriate time Facilitate any biopsies requested
Communications	Participate in surgical time out with OR and transplant teams Maintain contact with OPO and transplant centers regarding case progress Coordinate communication among OPO, transplant centers and UNOS regarding organ acceptance and/or declination
Documentation	Review all UNOS required documentation with surgeons, to include: ABO, brain death notes, infectious disease testing results Note times for actions such as: enter OR, first incision, cross-clamp, and exit OR Ensure all UNOS organ anatomy notation requirements are met
Organ Packaging and Labeling	Utilize Transnet (UNOS labeling system) to pack and label all organs and vessels Ensure UNOS requirements for triple sterile barriers for each organ are met Obtain all required Tissue typing materials such as: blood, nodes, spleen
Transportation	Collaborate with transplant teams to coordinate any needed surgical team transportation logistics before, during and after the surgical recovery Coordinate the transportation of any organs post recovery, as indicated

Follow-up Activities

Post-surgical recovery, the OPO performs a broad range of follow-up activities, including confirming the disposition of all organs which have been recovered for transplant and documenting those results in UNet [2]. Additionally, the OPO follows pending cultures associated with the donor case until all results are final, and reports positive results in a timely manner to any program which has transplanted an organ from the donor [2, 6, 8].

Each OPO has protocols in place for post-surgical recovery communications with donor families and the provision of ongoing support services tailored to meet family needs. Aftercare support programs for families are hallmarks of OPOs in demonstrating respect, sensitivity and gratitude to donors and their families. These protocols generally follow guidelines such as those published by the National Kidney Foundation (NKF) in their national donor family communication guidelines [10]. Program specific protocols also outline the OPO's communications with donor hospitals to facilitate the payment of all donation related expenses incurred [6, 8] and to provide a venue for feedback and process improvement initiatives. Additionally, OPOs and transplant programs facilitate joint venues to review and analyze clinical and quality metrics and to address any areas that merit process improvements or revisions [2, 3, 6, 8].

CONCLUSION

Professional relationships among transplant centers, donor hospitals and OPOs are essential to ensuring that the organs for which authorization has been so generously provided are matched efficiently, optimally, and safely to waiting recipients. Teamwork and collaboration among these organizations are hallmarks of the organ donation process. OPO policies and protocols, developed in adherence with all applicable laws, regulations, and standards, set the framework for meeting the goal of providing every eligible waiting recipient with a life-saving transplant. Through these coordinated efforts, and the provision of comprehensive and supportive donor family services, OPOs best honor the gift of organ donation so generously given by donors and their families.

CONSENT FOR PUBLICATION

Not applicable.

CONFLICT OF INTEREST

The author declares no conflict of interest, financial or otherwise.

ACKNOWLEDGEMENTS

Declared none.

REFERENCES

[1]   National Institutes of Health. National Organ Transplant Act; PUBLIC LAW 98-507-OCT 1984. Available from: https://history.nih.gov/research/downloads/PL98-507.pdf. [Accessed 1st April 2018]

[2]   U.S. Department of Health & Human Services Organ Procurement and Transplantation Network (OPTN) Policies Available from: https://optn.transplant.hrsa.gov/governance/policies/. [Accessed 4th April 2018]

[3]   Centers for Medicare and Medicaid Services. Conditions for Coverage (CfCs) & Conditions of Participations (CoPs) Available from: https://www.cms.gov/Regulations-and-Guidance/Legislation/CFCsAndCoPs/index.html?redirect=/cfcsandcops/16_asc.asp. [Accessed 1st April 2018]

[4]   Herdman R, Potts J. Non-Heart-Beating Organ Transplantation: Medical and Ethical Issues in Procurement Available from: https://www.nap.edu/read/ 6036/chapter/1 [Accessed 2nd April 2018]

[5]   The National Conference of Commissioners on Uniform State Laws. Uniform Anatomical Gift Act 2006. Available from: http://www.uniformlaws.org/Act.aspx?title=Anatomical%20Gift%20Act [Accessed 11th April 11 2018]

[6]   Association of Organ Procurement Organizations Organ Procurement Organization (OPO) Services Available from: http://www.aopo.org/about-opos/opo-programs/ [Accessed 11th April 2018]

[7]   The Living Legacy Foundation of Maryland. Clinical training programs Available from: https://www.thellf.org/ [Accessed 11th April 11 2018]

[8]   The Living Legacy Foundation of Maryland. Standard Operating Procedures Available from: https://www.thellf.org/ [Accessed 12th April 11 2018]

[9]   Rudon L, Ohler L, Shafer T. A Clinician's Guide to Donation and Transplantation. Lenexa, KS: Applied Measurements Professionals, Inc. 2006.

[10]   The National Kidney Foundation. Regarding Communication Among: Donor Families, Transplant Candidates/Recipients, Health Care Professionals Available from: https://www.kidney.org/transplantation/donorfamilies/infoPolicyGuidelines [Accessed 11th April 2018]

CHAPTER 3

Identification of the Brain Dead Donor

Justin Zamoyski and **Diana Greene-Chandos**[*]

The Ohio State University, Columbus, OH, USA

Abstract: The determination of brain death criteria has been the cornerstone of organ donation since 1968 when the Ad Hoc Committee at Harvard established medical definitions. It continues to stand the test of time as a means to establish medical and legal criteria for all transplant professionals in the field to rely upon and maintain the public's trust in the organ procurement system. This chapter reviews the origins of these criteria as well as the current application of neurologic criteria to determine brain death. It further reviews updated guidelines from the neurological professional community affirming these criteria and conduct of the brain death determination.

Keywords: Brain Dead Donor, Organ Donation, Organ Procurement, Transplantation Ethics.

INTRODUCTION

The history between brain death, with the recent preferred term of "death by neurological criteria" and organ donation has been intertwined ever since the first case reports in 1956 [1]. The first of the large committees to assess the determination of death by neurological criteria, the CIBA Symposium delineated the ethics of transplantation after the pronouncement of this type of death [2]. Within this symposium, the separation between patient care team and transplant team was first delineated. This dichotomy is the foundation for most institutional guidelines of the primary team notifying their organ procurement agency and not directly discussing organ donation with the patient's family. While addressed, the ethical concern over conflicts of interest remain to this day and it is important for the physicians involved in the declaration of death by neurological criteria to be knowledgeable in the specifics of the examination, limitations of the examination and additional ancillary testing as well as the legal aspects and special circumstances that can arise. This chapter will speak to all of these aspects.

[*] **Corresponding author Diana Greene-Chandos:** The Ohio State University, Columbus, OH, USA;
Tel: 3366923839; Emails: Diana.Greene-Chandos@osumc.edu; chandosfamily@gmail.com

Robert S.D. Higgins & Juan A. Sanchez (Eds.)

Understanding the ethics behind procurement after death by neurological criteria is hinged on understanding the evolution that there is a way to die other than circulatory arrest. In the setting of large brain injury, a detailed neurological examination will delineate coma from concern for meeting the criteria of death neurologically. In the first case series, brain death was considered a variant of coma being called "Le Coma Dépassé" [2]. This "irretrievable" coma was added to the end of the coma spectrum but as testing improved, it became a separate diagnosis [3]. This distinction gives specific scope to the examination in that it does not provide prognostic value like the Glasgow Coma Scale [4, 5] but rather indicates a specific diagnosis of death separate from cardiac death where there is no chance of recovery.

The examination itself has undergone relatively minimal changes due to the physiology tested. Changes to the criteria were primarily made to ensure the highest sensitivity and specificity available. Starting with the 1968 Ad Hoc Harvard Committee [3], the Schwab triad of unresponsive pupils, absence of spontaneous respirations and isoelectric EEG [6] were joined with other features to result in the Harvard Criteria. The final criteria added unresponsitivity and absent cranial nerve reflexes to the exam while also delineated timing of repeat testing at 24 hours with normothermia and absence of CNS depressants to improve the quality of testing [7]. These criteria were used in the only prospective study for brain death in 1977 by the NIH to try and develop further guideline changes. The study's primary endpoint was cardiac arrest after three months with supportive care. Of the 503 patients involved in the study, 19 met the Harvard Criteria and all suffered from cardiac arrest meaning that there was a high specificity but low sensitivity. By removing cranial nerve reflexes and only focusing on coma, apnea and flat EEG, they were able to include 189 patients in which 187 resulted in cardiac arrest with 2 patients having intoxication confounders. There were some limitations to the study in that consistency of cranial nerve reflex testing was varied and apnea testing was only of three minutes in duration due to concern for further brain damage [7].

With the data present in 1981, the President's Commission for the Study of Ethical Problems in Medicine and Biomedical and Behavioral Research released the briefly titled report "Defining Death" [8]. As per the report, the meaning of death consisted of irreversible cessation of circulatory and respiratory function while also including irreversible cessation of all functions of the entire brain including brainstem. This led to the Uniform Determination of Death Act in which the declaration of death proceeded in the same fashion for brain death or cardiac death. With a deceased patient as per these definitions, the physician is protected from criminal and civil liability while removing the patient from life support devices [9]. The exceptions to this occur in New York and New Jersey where the primary team are required to honor religious objections of the patient or their family [10, 11].

In 1995, the American Academy of Neurology set out to enhance the guidelines to further focus on refining the examination performed, eliminating clinical mimics for brain death and standardization of the apnea test [12]. The guidelines set forth, are similar to that which will be discussed later in the chapter with minimal change. In 2010, the AAN updated the guidelines. Based on the subsequent cases over those fifteen years, there was no data to invalidate the 1995 guidelines and no recoveries in adults had been reported [13]. These findings were reaffirmed in 2014 by the AAN.

PATHOLOGY AND PHYSIOLOGY

While brain death may be unique to the neurologic intensive care unit, it is hardly an uncommon one. In a prospective study of European intensive care units, brain death incidence was approximately 8% of ICU admissions compared to 20% for cardiopulmonary arrests not responding to resuscitation. This did not include withdrawal or withholding of care which accounted for 33% and 38% respectively which would have ultimately resulted in cessation of circulatory and respiratory functions [14].

While the initial pathology of injury may be variable, the mechanism of destruction remains consistent while progressing towards brain death. This mechanism is displacement of the thalamus and brainstem. The progression of this displacement will usually take place over the first few days as mass effect or edema will compress and eventually herniate the brainstem [15]. During the time that the patient is undergoing treatment for the primary pathology and sequelae, imminent brain death evaluations should be used. The two scales currently used are the Glasgow Coma scale and the Full Outline of Unresponsiveness or FOUR score. The GCS originally published in 1974 has diagnostic and prognostic value in patients with TBI by assessing motor function, verbal responsiveness and eye opening. While the most commonly used, it is frequently limited due to the intubation dependence affecting the verbal score of the assessment [4, 5]. The FOUR score uses motor function, eye opening, brainstem reflexes and respiratory pattern. Either system may be used by your institution since the corresponding outcomes were similarly accurate [16]. The lowest scores with GCS of 3 or FOUR score of 0 are both good indicators of impending brain death.

As the pathology progresses downwards, individual clinical features may evolve. Since the pathology most commonly originates in the thalamus, coma is an initial finding and progression inferiorly provides the brainstem findings in the brain death examination. Associated pituitary lesions will cause a loss of antidiuretic hormone in 75% of patients leading to neurogenic diabetes insipidus. The reason for variability is that a physiologic variant may have an extracranial blood supply for the pituitary and maintain some function. As damage extends to the pons, irregular breathing patterns will emerge such as Cheyne Stokes breathing. Extension to the medulla will cause a cessation of spontaneous breaths. Lesions in the rostral ventral neurons will lead to hypotension [17].

PREPARATION FOR CLINICAL EXAM

Prior to performing brain death testing, multiple clinical evaluations must be made to rule out clinical mimics of brain death. The assessments are meant to identify the patients from the NIH study who met prior criteria but did not actually have brain death [7].

Coma

Whether coma is caused by ischemic stroke, hemorrhage, anoxic injury, mass effect, edema or traumatic injury the cause must be established and found to be irreversible. This is established by optimal medical and surgical intervention of the primary pathology and sequelae of elevated intracranial pressure or hydrocephalus. While this treatment is being performed, exclusion of sedation or paralysis can be performed. Extra attention should be paid if the patient has been transferred due to possible loss in reporting. Due to this potential confounding factor, it may not be fruitful to perform brain death examination on admission [12, 13].

Neuroimaging Correlates

Having a primary pathology noted and treated does not obfuscate the need for evaluating for further confounders. Imaging should not just show pathology but pathology that is consistent with examination. TBI findings consistent with brain death would show multiple contusions or hematomas and shift of septum pellucidum from midline. Edema at the degree of causing brain death would be expected to have effacement of the basal cistern. Repeat imaging is encouraged if examination is still not consistent with scans to assess for evolution of primary lesions [12, 13].

Sedation Absent

When first seeing the patient, intoxication can be ruled out from available history and urine or serum toxicology screens. If patient has received any sedation in the healthcare setting, levels should be taken to ensure metabolism. While most guidelines accept the calculation of five half-lives as an alternative to serum levels if not readily attainable, those calculations assume normothermia with adequate hepatic and renal clearance. In the setting of hypothermia, sedation may take twice as long to clear given adequate pharmacodynamics [12, 13]. If pentobarbital has been used, the level must be measured as less than 10 µg/mL [12, 13, 20]. If ethanol is present, the level must be less than 80 mg/dL [12, 13].

Paralytic Absent

Most paralytic medications do not have readily available serum levels. To rule out paralysis as a confounding factor a train of four is needed. Using maximal impulse at the ulnar nerve should provide four out of four twitches. Deep tendon reflexes being present may also exclude neuromuscular blockade [18].

Absence of Metabolic Abnormalities

Frank changes in pH do not appear to have direct effects on the neurological examination. They indicate either an ongoing medical process that may limit examination or persistent toxicity. Metabolic acidosis may be secondary to cardiopulmonary arrest, sepsis or seizures which would indicate further treatment or evaluation for end organ damage may be necessary. An increased anion gap may also result from multiple ingestions including ethanol, methanol, ethylene glycol, acetaminophen, salicylates, cyanide, and cocaine. Respiratory acidosis would indicate ethanol, opiates, benzodiazepines or barbiturates. Correction is recommended for pH less than 7.20. While patient may be hyperventilated as part of treatment for elevated intracranial pressure, the $PaCO_2$ and pH should be normalized so as not to limit efficacy of the apnea test. While electrolytes are maintained closely in the intensive care unit, sodium levels may be elevated due to hypertonic therapy and the diabetes insipidus that will evolve from worsening injury. Sodium levels should be between 130- 160 mmol/L [12, 13].

Normothermia

Hypothermia limits examination on two different fronts. As the temperature declines, brainstem function declines as well. Most reflexes are resistant to hypothermia but may decline under 27°C and found to be completely absent below 20°C. While we may use hypothermia to lower the metabolic needs of the brain, it may also lower the metabolic production of the body as well. Since metabolism has been decreased, the production of carbon dioxide has decreased and will limit the effectiveness of the apnea test since it relies on carbon dioxide production at a specific level [19]. The recommended temperature to proceed with the examination is 36°C. For the examination to be the one determining death by neurological criteria, the temperature must be corrected to above this level through surface warming, warm intravenous fluids or targeted temperature devices [12, 13].

Normotension

As injury progresses and intracranial pressure increases, maintaining cerebral perfusion is key in management and ensuring normotension during testing is an important goal. A goal systolic blood pressure greater than 100mmHg is a reasonable goal to ensure cerebral perfusion and systemic organ perfusion during treatment and testing. This task may provide difficulty considering that diabetes insipidus may cause loss of vessel tone. Pressor support is recommended and no single pressor is preferred. It may be beneficial to have pressors available during examination due to the change of hypotension during the apnea test may cause premature termination [12, 13]. These authors prefer to augment the blood pressure to a systolic value of greater than 130mmHg immediately prior to apnea testing to ensure adequate perfusion throughout the apnea period.

Absence of Spontaneous Respirations

As an indicator of medullary damage, the absence of spontaneous respirations is necessary to proceed to brain death testing but not sufficient in diagnosing apnea. There are occasions where volume triggers for ventilation may be triggered by abdominal movements or cardiac excursion so it is recommended to place patient on pressure trigger to prevent auto-cycling [12, 13].

COMPONENTS OF BRAIN DEATH EXAMINATION

While assessing function after significant injury, localizing deficits is important in differentiating coma from brain death. There are aspects of the examination that look to the cortical and subcortical structures and aspects that focus on the reflex arcs within the brainstem circuitry. The most critical first step is to ascertain the degree of consciousness and before continuing forward with the examination, the patient must be unconscious without any response to voice or noxious stimuli. The next segment is to determine the degree of physical movement with noxious stimuli of the extremities. The resultant purposeful movement, reflexive movement or lack of any movement will determine localization of dysfunction of the cortical and/or subcortical structures. These will be specifically discussed below. The next component of the examination is cranial nerve testing. It is easiest to work cephalad to caudad regarding the reflexes of the brainstem to ensure no reflexes are missed [12, 13]. Each reflex is discussed below separately. When communicating findings, it may be helpful to use 'reflex absent' or 'reflex present' instead of positive or negative due to the variability of the latter's usage.

Pupillary Reflexes

This test focuses on cranial nerves II and III, the most cephalad of the cranial nerves with nuclei in the midbrain. The test is performed by opening both eyes and shining a light in each eye, looking for contraction of the pupillary muscle and decrease in diameter size of the pupil. In the patient dead by neurological criteria, pupils are mid-size measuring four to six millimeters and are non-reactive to light (Fig. **3.1**). The pupils may be larger due to intact thoracic sympathetic input being unopposed by the cranial nerve III's parasympathetic signal. Most forms of sedation will cause meiosis but not affect the reactivity of the pupil. Some paralytics, especially atracurium and vecuronium have been found to limit the reactivity to light [21]. If there is any reactivity to light, then this reflex is considered present and the patient should not undergo further examination for death by neurological criteria [13, 14]. If there is concern as to whether reactivity is present by use of a pen light, then a more accurate measurement of pupillary reactivity can occur with use of a pupilometer [22].

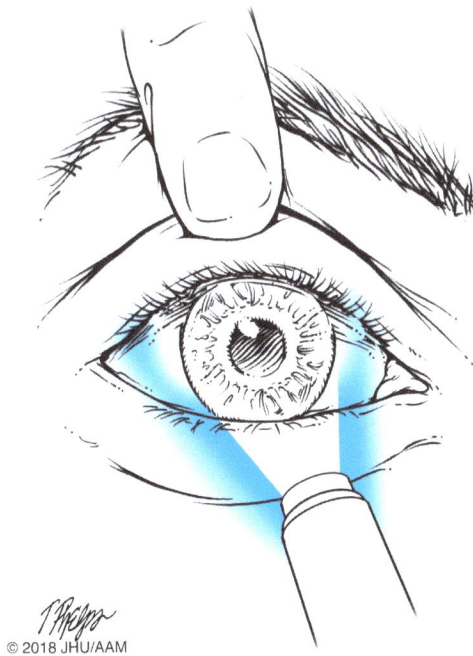

© 2018 JHU/AAM

Fig. (3.1). Mid-size pupils showing no reactivity to pen-light examination. Medical Illustrations© 2018 Tim Phelps, MS, FAMI, Johns Hopkins University.

Corneal Reflexes

Testing cranial nerves V and VII can be performed with either a cotton swab or squirting water onto the cornea of the eye while held open. Any activity of closing the eyelid of contraction of the orbicularis oculi would be interpreted as the reflex being present and would be <u>not consistent</u> with death by neurological criteria. No movement of the eyelid would be interpreted as the reflex being absent. Two items are important for accurate testing of this reflex. The first is that the eyes not be held open too forcefully as it can limit the ability to visualize a subtle blink or contraction. The second is to be certain that the area of the cornea is being touched. This is the area over the iris of the eye. If the sclera (the area that is mostly over the white of the eye) is touched, it likely will not elucidate a response leading to false evaluation [13, 14].

Oculocephalic Reflex

Cervical spine clearance must be obtained prior to proceeding with part of the examination. While testing cranial nerves III, IV and VI you will need to hold the eyes open and rotate the patients head horizontally. Absence of this reflex will present as the eyes remaining straight in relation to the head and not undergoing rapid movement towards their prior location (Fig. **3.2**). A common error is slow rotation of the head which may not stimulate the vestibular system enough to initiate the reflex. The resting gaze may be slightly divergent or skewed but assessment can still be performed. Any movement of the eyes including saccades indicates that there is brainstem activity and is <u>not consistent</u> with brain death [13, 14].

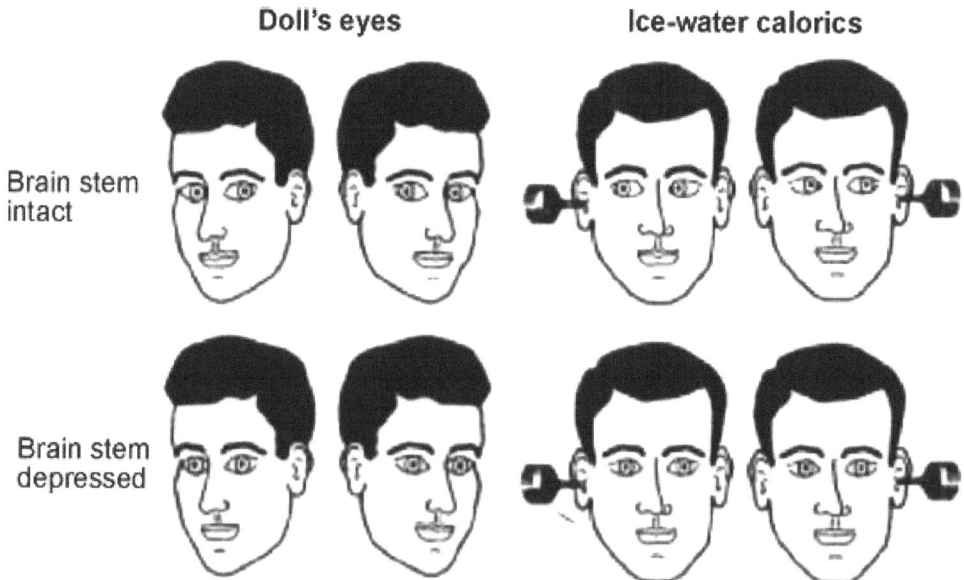

Fig. (3.2). This shows the oculocephalic reflex (Doll's eyes) in column one and the oculovestibular reflex (ice-water calorics) in column two. The depictions in the "brainstem depressed" row are what should be seen in both reflexes when declaring death by neurological criteria. From Merchut and Biller, Neupsy Key, 2016 [24]. Medical Illustrations© 2018 Tim Phelps, MS, FAMI, Johns Hopkins University.

Oculovestibular Reflex

While the oculocephalic reflex utilizes activation of the vestibular system, it does not utilize the nucleus of cranial nerve VIII. The oculovestibular reflex focuses on the function of cranial nerve VIII and the resultant effects on cranial nerves III and VI with eye movements that are observed. Elevating the head of bed to thirty degrees will place the horizontal canal in the vertical position, optimizing its response and resulting eye movements. While applying sixty milliliters of ice cold water, the endolymph of the horizontal canal will undergo sedimentation activating the eyes to slowly move towards the stimulated ear with saccades in the opposing direction when the reflex is intact and present (Fig. **3.2**). While any movement is <u>not consistent</u> with brain death, it may be prudent to place marks on the lower lids to ensure no movements can been seen given that holding open the eyes may confound interpretation of movement. After finishing injection, monitor for one minute to ensure no activation has taken place. It is recommended to wait five minutes before testing the other side as there may be suppression from stimulus in the opposing vestibular system. Although all ocular reflexes have confounders of trauma, edema of the lids or globes, the oculovestibular reflex has unique confounders that must be evaluated such as cerumen in the external auditory canal and battle sign since basilar fracture may provide unilateral findings. It also requires an intact tympanic membrane; therefore, it is imperative to view the membrane with an otoscope prior to starting this reflex [13, 14].

Facial Noxious Stimuli

This test may be considered part of the noxious stimuli assessing for coma but it does focus on the nuclei for cranial nerves V and VII. Pressure may be applied to either the supraorbital foramens inducing signal along the V1 distribution or the condyles of the temporal-mandibular joint activating V3. Any activation of the facial muscles is <u>not consistent</u> with death by neurological criteria [12, 13].

Pharyngeal and Tracheal Reflexes

Cough and gag reflexes are often grouped together because they involve the same cranial nerves. A strong reason why both should be tested is the unreliability of gag in patients who are currently intubated due to possible refractory response from cranial nerves IX and X. Gag should be performed by tongue depressor stimulation of the posterior oropharynx. Cough reflex can be tested by applying the suction catheter through the endotracheal tube and suctioning for several seconds. Another test that can be used for cranial nerve X is atropine injection. Administration that fails to cause tachycardia indicates vagal dysfunction. This testing may not be included in institutional guidelines and was not included in the 1995 AAN guidelines and every updated guideline since then [12, 13].

Noxious Stimuli in Extremities

While functionally this part of the exam assesses coma pathology in the upper brain, it is the last part of the clinical exam per the systematic approach. This can be tested by nail bed pressure on the fingers of the upper extremities and toes of the lower extremities. Sternal Rubbing or rib rubbing in the axilla are not commonly accepted as appropriate tests for a death examination. In addition, areola twisting, is never accepted as means for noxious stimulation in any situation. When performing these tests, it is important to identify withdrawal or posturing from lower extremity spinal mediated reflexes which are still consistent with brain death. Any movement of the upper extremities to noxious stimuli is considered <u>not consistent</u> with death by neurological criteria. However, in the lower extremities, a triple flexion response with flexion of the ankle, knee and hip briskly followed by quick relaxation is a response considered entirely spinal and is considered acceptable to see and still call <u>consistent</u> with death by neurological criteria. If any movement of the leg other than this occurs then this would be considered <u>not consistent </u>with death by neurological criteria [12, 13]. As one can imagine, this can cause consternation and confusion in the families of the patient. Therefore, these authors typically prepare the family before the examination occurs, that this movement can be seen and is entirely mediated from the lower spine only. Twitching of the trunk muscles including pectoralis and abdominal can be seen in ischemia of the anterior horns of the spinal cord and are acceptable to see and still declare death [25].

APNEA TESTING

The apnea test is also called the apneic oxygenation-diffusion test, and it is the most common evaluation of respiratory drive evaluating the ventral and dorsal respiratory groups which span the entire length of the medulla. Preoxygenation is recommended with 100% of FiO_2 even if the patient is saturating well because the removal of nitrogen stores will facilitate oxygen transportation during the examination and prevent aborting the apnea test due to dropping saturations [26].

Further preparation for the apnea test is similar to the clinical examination. Normothermia, normotension and normocapnea should be maintained with resources available to ensure maximal safety for the patient and integrity of testing. Hypothermia may decrease metabolism of the tissues leading to depressed carbon dioxide production and may also cause an oxyhemoglobin shift to the left resulting in decreased oxygen delivery to tissues. Hypotension is avoided for similar oxygen delivery concerns which may damage organs that qualify for transplantation should the patient wishes to be a donor. Pressor support may be used in either continuous drip or phenylephrine injection to ensure appropriate perfusion. If there are hypoxic or hypotensive concerns, stability at a PEEP of 5cm H_2O may indicate tolerance of cannula placement for testing. Normocapnea with $PaCO_2$ of 35-45mmHg should be obtained so that patient will develop appropriate respiratory drive. The one exception to this is in the patient with COPD associated CO_2 retention, where the $PaCO_2$ should be at the level that is typical for the patient [27].

After pre-oxygenation the ventilator should be disconnected and a cannula with six liters per minute of oxygen should be placed down the ET tube 1 cm beyond the end to ensure proper placement above the carina. For the first few minutes' oxygen saturation should be monitored closely to prevent complications from mal-positioning or trauma [27]. In a study of 212 apnea tests, only 3% were not completed mainly due to hypotension. Mean PaO_2 during these tests remained relative stable decreasing from 265mmHg to 236mmHg, indicating appropriate oxygen delivery [28].

During apnea, ensuring the patient is apneic is rather important. Visually observing for chest expansion, clavicle elevation or abdominal excursion may show activity which is not consistent with brain death and apnea testing should be aborted. The chest and abdomen may have slight excursions from the heartbeat and if synchronous with pulse, should be monitored while apnea test can continue [27].

At normal temperature, the $PaCO_2$ in an apneic patient is expected to raise 3-6mmHg per minute [29]. An ABG should be obtained 8 minutes into the examination. It is important to be able to obtain the arterial blood sample quickly ideally through a functioning arterial line. In circumstances where no arterial line is in place, please allow for time to obtain the sample and prepare to sample it from a place likely to be the easiest to access which is the femoral artery in most cases. Once the ABG is obtained, remove the cannula and place the patient back on the ventilator. The $PaCO_2$ should rise more than 20mmHg, and if the patient is normocapneic at beginning of exam, it should have an endpoint $PaCO_2$ of 60mmHg or greater which is <u>consistent</u> with death by neurological criteria. If the apnea test is <u>consistent</u> with neurological criteria, time of death is pronounced when results of the ABG are interpreted [27]. Severe increase in $PaCO_2$ and the resulting decrease in pH may cause cardiovascular instability which may put donor organs at risk [28, 30]. Continuous carbon dioxide monitoring has been used in some institutions to prevent overproduction of carbon dioxide although no guidelines for this exist currently [30].

The main endpoint for apnea testing is eight minutes of duration which should provide the appropriate amount of time for results <u>consistent</u> with death by neurological criteria should it be the case [27]. Apnea testing should be aborted if any respirations are seen, systolic blood pressure drops below 90mmHg, new cardiac arrhythmias or oxygen desaturation less than 85% persists longer than 30 seconds [28, 30]. When an apnea needs to be aborted, a blood gas should be rapidly obtained, if possible, to determine if $PaCO_2$ has increased by more than 20mmHg or a final value of more than 60mmHg to be consistent with death. If $PaCO_2$ is less than those values then it is <u>not consistent</u> with death by neurological criteria and apnea testing may be repeated for ten minutes if patient can tolerate it [27, 28, 30].

Though recommended by the current guidelines, apnea testing has come under recent discussion in the realm of organ transplant. There have been no case reports that a patient whose clinical exam is consistent with brain death but the patient has spontaneous respirations can recover to a level of coma better than their current state [30]. A patient with this clinical picture is then required to undergo organ donation after cardiac death compared to brain death which limits organs that may be procured. Another point of contention is that low oxygen delivery during the apnea test from hypotension or hypoxia, although rare, may cause harm to organs rendering them unsuitable for transplant [28, 30]. This, however, needs to be balanced with the certainty provided with such testing, that in these authors opinions, often is enough for families who are skeptical of death occurring in this way, once they see that no attempt to breathe in 8 min has occurred.

Apnea testing, as described above, in patients on extracorporeal membrane oxygenation (ECMO) is not possible as gas exchange occurs entirely through the membrane oxygenator. However, there have been multiple published case-reports, case series, and reviews on how to appropriately assess the apnea reflex in patients on ECMO. It has not yet been elevated to the point of reaching national guidelines, but is worth mentioning as the protocol being used has been consistent. Talahma and Degeorgia provide a step-wise approach in their review with the following [31]:

Adjust the sweep rate at the ECMO to achieve normocapnia ($PaCO_2$ of 35-45 mmHg).

Perform 10 minutes of pre-oxygenation by increasing the FiO_2 of the oxygenator on the ECMO machine to 100%.

Disconnect the patient from the ventilator and place a cannula through endotracheal tube to the level of the carina running 100% oxygen at a rate of 5-8 L/min.

Maintain the same ECMO settings including the flow rate and FiO_2 but gradually decrease the gas sweep rate to as low as 0.5 L/min as tolerated by the patient.

Watch for any sign of respiratory effort.

Repeat the ABG after 5 minutes and then again after 10 minutes.

If the required $PaCO_2$ level (> 60 mmHg or an Δ increase of 20 mmHg) is not achieved after 10 minutes and the patient remains hemodynamically stable, continue the low gas sweep for another 5 min. and repeat the ABG.

The apnea test is considered <u>consistent</u> with death by neurological criteria if no respiratory movements are seen and the arterial $PaCO_2$ is greater than 60mmHg and increased by 20mmHg over the baseline $PaCO_2$.

ANCILLARY TESTING

The use of ancillary testing varies among countries and institutions. Since the 1995 AAN guidelines there have been no distinctions as to a preferred test and the only recommendation is that testing be performed if components of the exam cannot be evaluated consistently. In the 2010 guidelines, it is recommended that ancillary testing only be performed if and only if a complete examination with apnea test cannot be completed in its entirety as it has remained the most reliable evaluation to date. Nonetheless, reliable ancillary testing does become important when aspects of the exam cannot be complete especially in the setting trauma to the orbits and face limiting reflex testing or when the apnea test cannot be complete. The tests available fall into two different categories: neurologic function and blood flow [12, 13].

Electrophysiological Testing

Historically EEG has been the primary ancillary test for brain death examination due to its wide availability. Prior to the Harvard Ad Hoc Committee, case reports had demonstrated that isoelectric EEGs had not been a reliable indicator of irreversible coma [3]. Further assessment by the President's Commission state the only outcome change of EEG in anoxic injury is decreased time of observation without any confounders that may alter it [8]. The same report also refers to another article which states that clinical findings consistent with brain death and non-isoelectric EEG have a prognosis that is "similarly hopeless" [32, 33]. There are other limitations to EEG in an ICU setting due to electrical equipment interfering with the strict criteria for isoelectric readings but with clinical examination has been seen to have sensitivity and specificity over 90% [34]. Listed below are the minimal guideline for EEG recording when testing for electrocerebral silence from the AAN guidelines of 2010 [13].

- Minimum of eight scalp electrodes
- Interelectrode dependencies should be between 100 and 10,000
- Integrity of the entire recording system should be tested
- Electrode distances should be at least 10 cm Sensitivity should be increased to at least 2 μV for 30 minutes with inclusion of appropriate calibrations
- High-frequency filter setting should be at 30 Hz, and low-frequency setting should not be below 1 Hz
- There should be no electroencephalographic reactivity to intense somatosensory or audiovisual stimuli

In addition to the sixteen channels EEG the use of evoked potentials has also been available. Evoked potentials have the advantage of remaining present in comatose state but absent in brain death. Auditory evoked potentials do have the limitation of only activating the pons and not the medulla. Somatosensory evoked potentials may have clinical benefit but since the 1995 guidelines have had limited data [12].

Vascular Imaging

Due to improvement of technology there are several modalities for imaging vascular flow. Transcranial Doppler (TCD) has had multiple studies and is shown to have sensitivity of 91% and specificity of 100%. There is a specific pattern of flow in brain death that can exclude focal lesions to the brain stem [34, 35]. The biggest limiting factor is technique and experience which continues to improve. Magnetic resonance angiography (MRA) and computed tomography angiography (CTA) may be used but validity has not been sufficiently tested per the 2010 AAN guideline update [13]. Nuclear scintigraphy may be used with portable gamma camera so that patient can stay in the ICU. A study that is consistent with death by neurological criteria will present with a specific image showing no uptake in intracranial arteries but around the skull creating an "empty lightbulb" sign or there may be uptake in the nose creating a "hot nose" sign (Fig. **3.3**). Nuclear brain scanning correlates to TCD and CTA [38]. The final vascular imaging is the most invasive with a four vessel cerebral angiogram (Fig. **3.4**). While there was concern that the pressure injections may falsely create flow, most observations have shown that the low resistance cerebral arteries develop high resistance and will have no flow to contrast injection. With this imaging contrast can also be given at the aortic arch which will create a pattern of contrast tracking upwards but stopping at the petrous carotid. You can also see the vertebral arteries filling with flow stopping upon entry to the skull as well. Despite these concerns, cerebral angiography remains the gold standard for ancillary testing when declaring death by neurological criteria [36, 37].

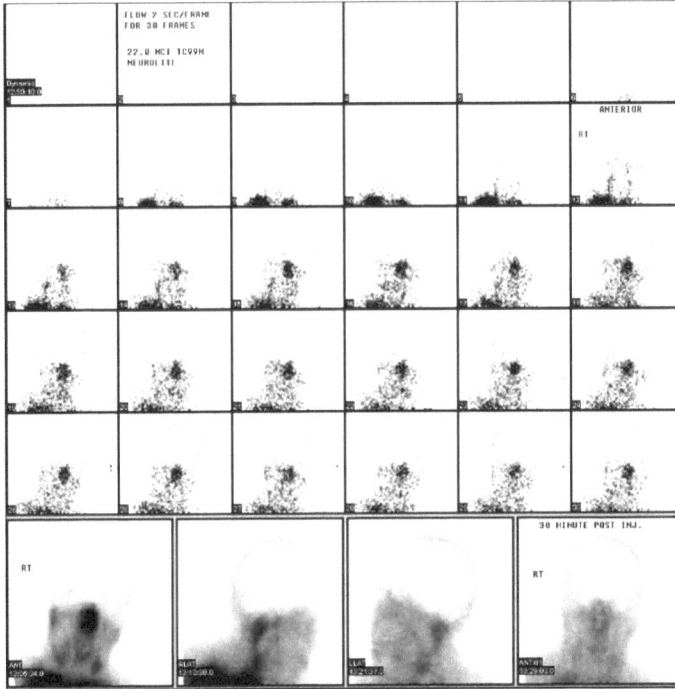

Fig. (3.3). Example of cerebral nuclear scintigraphy <u>consistent</u> with death by neurological criteria. The area of the brain shows no uptake but does show the "hot nose" sign. JasonRobertYoungMD, CC BY-SA 4.0 (image not altered) [42]. Medical Illustrations© 2018 Tim Phelps, MS, FAMI, Johns Hopkins University.

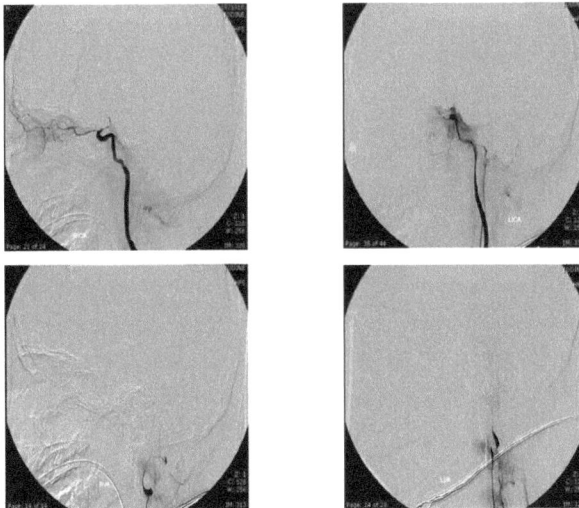

Fig. (3.4). Clockwise from top left these images show cerebral angiography injections from the right internal carotid artery (ICA), left ICA, left vertebral artery (VA) and right VA. As shown there no flow into the intracranial cavity from any of the vessels, making this angiogram <u>consistent </u>with death by neurological criteria [23]. Medical Illustrations© 2018 Tim Phelps, MS, FAMI, Johns Hopkins University.

SPECIAL CIRCUMSTANCES

Pediatric Patients

While the timing of the process of declaration death by neurological criteria in adults, in terms of number of examinations, time between examinations and number of certifying varies based on state statutes and institutional guidelines, the pediatric patients process definitions are more specific. All pediatric patients are recommended to have two examinations, along with two apnea tests. The time between examinations has been set at 24 hours for neonates up until 30 days after birth, and 12 hours for those children from 1 month of age to 18 years of age. The time between exams may be abbreviated with the use of an ancillary test. Children over the age of 14 being managed in an adult trauma ICU may be diagnosed using adult guidelines, in keeping with existing hospital policies [23].

"Brainstem" Death

There remains some philosophical debate as to whether or not brainstem death in the circumstance of primary brainstem destruction (*i.e.* typically from a primary brainstem hemorrhage) is truly whole brain death [40]. The United Kingdom recognizes brainstem death as death and only refers to death by neurological criteria as brainstem death. Germany, on the other hand, requires that a confirmatory test be performed showing no cortical activity with their stance being that the bedside neurological examination is only accurately testing the brainstem and not the cortical responses [41]. The AAN guidelines do not differentiate between brain or brainstem death [12, 13]. However, each state in the United States has laws which can dictate how many examinations should occur and how often as well as whether the declaration requires two separate professional evaluations. Many states use the language of "acceptable medical standards" as to how death by neurological criteria is determined [39].

Maternal Death by Neurological Criteria

While this is a rare circumstance, it is one of note does pose an ethical quandary worth considering. Current standards of care are that most will support the mother's cardiopulmonary system with a greater than a 16 week old fetus for as long as possible until the fetus is 28 weeks then will deliver. There are 30 documented infants born in this way who initially had low Apgar scores but achieved normal developmental milestones [40].

Religious Exceptions

Most major religions of the world are accepting of death by neurological criteria.

However, there are two that clearly do not recognize death is this way and that includes persons from the Orthodox Jewish faith and Shinto religion of Japan (Fig. **3.5**). In the United States, at the moment, there are only two states, New York and New Jersey, that recognize religious exception as a reason to not accept death by neurological criteria [40].

Symbol	✝	✡	☪	☸	水	ॐ	⛩
Religion	Christian	Judaic	Islamic	Buddist	Confucian	Hindu	Shinto
Death by Neuro-logical Criteria	Accepted	Accept-ed by most Rabbis	Accept-ed	Accept-ed	Accepted	Accept-ed	Mostly Unaccept-able

Fig. (3.5). The positions on death by neurological criteria from some major religions of the world [40]. Medical Illustrations© 2018 Tim Phelps, MS, FAMI, Johns Hopkins University.

CONSENT FOR PUBLICATION

Not applicable.

CONFLICT OF INTEREST

The author declares no conflict of interest, financial or otherwise.

ACKNOWLEDGEMENTS

Declared none.

REFERENCES

[1]   Mollaret P, Goulon M. Le coma depasse (memoire preliminaire). Rev Neurol (Paris) 1959; 101: 3-15. [PMID: 14423403]

[2]   Murray JE. Organ transplantation: the practical possibilities. In: Wolstenholme GEW, O'Conner M, Eds. Ciba Foundation Symposium: Ethics in Medical Progress. 54-77.

[3]   A definition of irreversible coma. Report of the Ad Hoc Committee of the Harvard Medical School to Examine the Definition of Brain Death. JAMA 1968; 205(6): 337-40. [http://dx.doi.org/10.1001/jama.1968.03140320031009] [PMID: 5694976]

[4]   Choi SC, Barnes TY, Bullock R, Germanson TA, Marmarou A, Young HF. Temporal profile of outcomes in severe head injury. J Neurosurg 1994; 81(2): 169-73. [http://dx.doi.org/10.3171/jns.1994.81.2.0169] [PMID: 8027796]

[5]   Choi SC, Narayan RK, Anderson RL, Ward JD. Enhanced specificity of prognosis in severe head

injury. J Neurosurg 1988; 69(3): 381-5.
[http://dx.doi.org/10.3171/jns.1988.69.3.0381] [PMID: 3404236]

[6]   Schwab RS, Potts F, Mathis P. EEG as an aid in determining death in the presence of cardiac activity. Electroencephalogr Clin Neurophysiol 1963; 15: 147.

[7]   An appraisal of the criteria of cerebral death. A summary statement. A collaborative study. JAMA 1977; 237(10): 982-6.
[http://dx.doi.org/10.1001/jama.1977.03270370054022] [PMID: 576252]

[8]   Defining death: a report on the medical, legal, ethical issues in the determination of death Washinton. D.C.: Government Printing Office 1981.

[9]   National Conference of Commissioners on Uniform State Laws. 1981. The Uniform Determination of Death Act 1981. from www.uniformlaws.org/shared/docs/determination%20of%20death/udda80.pdf

[10]   New Jersey Office of the Attorney General. 2007. New Jersey register volume 39, issue 9, issue date: May 7, 2007. Rule adoptions law and public safety division of consumer affairs board of medical examiners. Adopted repeal and new rules: N.J.A.C. 13:35-6A. Declarations of death upon the basis of neurological criteria, from http://www.state.nj.us/oag/ca/adoption/bmeado57.htm

[11]   New York State Department of Health 2005. New York State Department of Health Guidelines for Determining Brain death, from http://www.health.state.ny.us/professionals/doctors/guidelines/ determination_of_brain_death/docs/determination_of_brain_death.pdf

[12]   Wijdicks EFM. Determining brain death in adults. Neurology 1995; 45(5): 1003-11.
[http://dx.doi.org/10.1212/WNL.45.5.1003] [PMID: 7746373]

[13]   Wijdicks EFM, Varelas PN, Gronseth GS, Greer DM. Evidence-based guideline update: determining brain death in adults: report of the Quality Standards Subcommittee of the American Academy of Neurology. Neurology 2010; 74(23): 1911-8.
[http://dx.doi.org/10.1212/WNL.0b013e3181e242a8] [PMID: 20530327]

[14]   Sprung CL, Cohen SL, Sjokvist P, *et al.* End-of-life practices in European intensive care units: the Ethicus Study. JAMA 2003; 290(6): 790-7.
[http://dx.doi.org/10.1001/jama.290.6.790] [PMID: 12915432]

[15]   Gerard RW. Anoxia and neural metabolism. Arch Neurol Psychiatry 1938; 20: 50-7.

[16]   Iyer VN, Mandrekar JN, Danielson RD, Zubkov AY, Elmer JL, Wijdicks EF. Validity of the FOUR score coma scale in the medical intensive care unit. Mayo Clin Proc 2009; 84(8): 694-701.
[http://dx.doi.org/10.4065/84.8.694] [PMID: 19648386]

[17]   Leestma JE, Hughes JR, Diamond ER. Temporal correlates in brain death. EEG and clinical relationships to the respirator brain. Arch Neurol 1984; 41(2): 147-52.
[http://dx.doi.org/10.1001/archneur.1984.04050140045021] [PMID: 6691814]

[18]   Kainuma M, Miyake T, Kanno T. Extremely prolonged vecuronium clearance in a brain death case. Anesthesiology 2001; 95(4): 1023-4.
[http://dx.doi.org/10.1097/00000542-200110000-00035] [PMID: 11605900]

[19]   Fischbeck KH, Simon RP. Neurological manifestations of accidental hypothermia. Ann Neurol 1981; 10(4): 384-7.
[http://dx.doi.org/10.1002/ana.410100411] [PMID: 7316491]

[20]   LaMancusa J, Cooper R, Vieth R, Wright F. The effects of the falling therapeutic and subtherapeutic barbiturate blood levels on electrocerebral silence in clinically brain-dead children. Clin Electroencephalogr 1991; 22(2): 112-7.
[http://dx.doi.org/10.1177/155005949102200212] [PMID: 2032344]

[21]   Shlugman D, Parulekar M, Elston JS, Farmery A. Abnormal pupillary activity in a brainstem-dead patient. Br J Anaesth 2001; 86(5): 717-20.
[http://dx.doi.org/10.1093/bja/86.5.717] [PMID: 11575350]

[22]   Larson MD, Muhiudeen I. Pupillometric analysis of the 'absent light reflex'. Arch Neurol 1995; 52(4): 369-72.
[http://dx.doi.org/10.1001/archneur.1995.00540280051018] [PMID: 7710372]

[23]   Souter MJ. Declaration of Brain Death 2013. http://www.aopo.org/wikidonor/declaration -of-bra-n-death/

[24]   Merchut MP, Biller J. Acute Loss of Consciousness in Neupsy Key https://neupsykey.com/assessment-of-acute-loss-of-consciousness/

[25]   Beckmann YY, Ciftçi Y, Seçil Y, Eren S. Fasciculations in brain death. Crit Care Med 2010; 38(12): 2377-8.
[http://dx.doi.org/10.1097/CCM.0b013e3181fa0458] [PMID: 20890193]

[26]   al Jumah M, McLean DR, al Rajeh S, Crow N. Bulk diffusion apnea test in the diagnosis of brain death. Crit Care Med 1992; 20(11): 1564-7.
[http://dx.doi.org/10.1097/00003246-199211000-00014] [PMID: 1424700]

[27]   Earnest MP, Beresford HR, McIntyre HB. Testing for apnea in suspected brain death: methods used by 129 clinicians. Neurology 1986; 36(4): 542-4.
[http://dx.doi.org/10.1212/WNL.36.4.542] [PMID: 3960329]

[28]   Goudreau JL, Wijdicks EFM, Emery SF. Complications during apnea testing in determination of brain death: predisposing factors. Neurology 2008; 70: 284-9.
[PMID: 18077794]

[29]   Eger EI, Severinghaus JW. The rate of rise of PaCO2 in the apneic anesthetized patient. Anesthesiology 1961; 22: 419-25.
[http://dx.doi.org/10.1097/00000542-196105000-00013] [PMID: 13725901]

[30]   Wijdicks EFM, Rabinstein AA, Manno EM, Atkinson JD. Pronouncing brain death: Contemporary practice and safety of the apnea test. Neurology 2008; 71(16): 1240-4.
[http://dx.doi.org/10.1212/01.wnl.0000327612.69106.4c] [PMID: 18852438]

[31]   Talahma M, Degorgia M. Apena testing for determination of brain death in patients supported by extracorporeal membrane oxygenation. J Neurol Res 2016; 6(1): 28-34.
[http://dx.doi.org/10.14740/jnr376w]

[32]   Chatrian GE. Electrophysiologic evaluation of brain death: a critical appraisal. Electrodiagnosis in Clinical Neurology. New York: Churchill Livingstone 1980.

[33]   Bennett DR, Korein J, Hughes JR, Merlis JK, Suter C. Atlas of electroencephalography in coma and cerebral death. New York: Raven Press 1976.

[34]   Grigg MM, Kelly MA, Celesia GG, Ghobrial MW, Ross ER. Electroencephalographic activity after brain death. Arch Neurol 1987; 44(9): 948-54.
[http://dx.doi.org/10.1001/archneur.1987.00520210048018] [PMID: 3619714]

[35]   Petty GW, Mohr JP, Pedley TA, *et al.* The role of transcranial Doppler in confirming brain death: sensitivity, specificity, and suggestions for performance and interpretation. Neurology 1990; 40(2): 300-3.
[http://dx.doi.org/10.1212/WNL.40.2.300] [PMID: 2405294]

[36]   Pearson J, Korein J, Braunstein P. Morphology of defectively perfused brains in patients with persistent extracranial circulation. Ann N Y Acad Sci 1978; 315: 265-71.
[http://dx.doi.org/10.1111/j.1749-6632.1978.tb50344.x] [PMID: 284738]

[37]   Kricheff II, Pinto RS, George AE, Braunstein P, Korein J. Angiographic findings in brain death. Ann N Y Acad Sci 1978; 315: 168-83.
[http://dx.doi.org/10.1111/j.1749-6632.1978.tb50338.x] [PMID: 284734]

[38]   Hazratji SM, Singh BM, Strobos RJ. Angiography in brain death. N Y State J Med 1981; 81(1): 82-3.
[PMID: 6936623]

[39]   Goodman JM, Heck LL, Moore BD. Confirmation of brain death with portable isotope angiography: a review of 204 consecutive cases. Neurosurgery 1985; 16(4): 492-7.
[PMID: 3990928]

[40]   Wijdicks EFM. Brain Death. 2nd ed., Oxford University Press 2011.

[41]   Wissenschaftlicher Beirat der Bundesärztekammer. Richtlinien zur Feststellung des Hirntodes. Dtsch Arztebl 1998; 53(39): A 1861-8.

[42]   Young JR. File:radionuclide cerebral blood flow scanpng 2015. CC BY-SA 4.0

CHAPTER 4

Management of Public Health Service (PHS) Increased Risk Donors and Hepatitis C or HIV Infected Donors

Nicole Theodoropoulos[*, 1], **Stephanie Pouch**[2] and **Dorry Segev**[3]

[1] *Division of Infectious Diseases & Immunology, University of Massachusetts, 55 Lake Avenue North, Worcester, MA, 01655, USA*

[2] *Division of Infectious Diseases, Emory University School of Medicine, Atlanta, GA, USA*

[3] *Johns Hopkins University School of Medicine, Baltimore, MD, USA*

Abstract: The goal of this chapter is to review the currently Public Health Service defined increased risk donors and discuss management of recipients of these donor organs.

Keywords: Hepatitis C Virus, HIV to HIV Transplantation, PHS Increased Risk Donors.

INTRODUCTION

In 1994, when HIV was still a relatively new and commonly fatal infection, the United States Public Health Service (PHS) released guidelines to define organ donors that should be excluded from donation due to concerns for undiagnosed HIV infection [1]. These guidelines were adopted by the Organ Procurement and Transplantation Network (OPTN) and eventually required Organ Procurement Organizations (OPOs) to classify donors with risk factors that, according to the PHS criteria, made them at a higher risk for acute infection with HIV, hepatitis B virus (HBV) and/or hepatitis C virus (HCV) and, therefore, a higher risk for infection undetected by routine screening tests, and concomitantly a higher risk for unintentional transmission of infection to organ recipients. The guidelines were updated in 2013 to reflect the substantial changes in HIV epidemiology and risks as well as to incorporate more specific data regarding the risk of acute HBV and HCV infection [2]. These guidelines are no longer considered exclusionary but are used to aid transplant centers in weighing risks and benefits when offering

[*] **Corresponding author Nicole Theodoropoulos:** Division of Infectious Diseases & Immunology, University of Massachusetts, 55 Lake Avenue North, Worcester, MA, 01655, USA; Fax: 5088565981; 5088563158; Email: nicole.theodoropoulos@umassmemorial.org

organs that are at increased risk for HIV, HBV and/or HCV transmission to transplant candidates (Table **4.1**). These donors were formerly referred to as "CDC high risk donors" but are currently termed as "PHS increased risk donors".

Table 4.1. Public Health Service Guidelines for Increased Risk Donor Designation.

1994 Guideline (All Ages)	2013 Guideline (All Ages)
Persons who have had sex in the preceding 12 months with any person described in items 1-4 or with a person known or suspected to have HIV infection	People who have had **sex with a person known or suspected to have HIV, HBV, or HCV** infections in the preceding 12 months
Men who have had sex with another man (MSM) in the preceding 5 yrs	**MSM** in the preceding 12 months
Persons who have had sex in the preceding 12 months with any person described in items 1-4 or with a person known or suspected to have HIV infection	Women who have had **sex with a man with a history of MSM** behavior in the preceding 12 months
Men and women who have engaged in sex in exchange for money or drugs in the preceding 5 years	People who have had **sex in exchange for money or drugs** in the preceding 12 months
Persons who have had sex in the preceding 12 months with any person described in items 1-4 or with a person known or suspected to have HIV infection	People who have had **sex with a person who had sex in exchange for money or drugs** in the preceding 12 months
Persons who have had sex in the preceding 12 months with any person described in items 1-4 or with a person known or suspected to have HIV infection	People who have had **sex with a person that has injected drugs** by IV, IM, or subcutaneous route for nonmedical reasons in the preceding 12 months
Persons who report nonmedical IV, IM, or subcutaneous injection of drugs in the preceding 5 years	People who have **injected drugs** by IV, IM, or subcutaneous route for nonmedical reasons in the preceding 12 months
Inmates of correctional systems.	People who have been in **lockup, jail, prison, or a juvenile correctional facility** for $\geq$ 72 hours in the preceding 12 months
Person who have history, physical exam, medical records, or autopsy reports reveal other evidence sexually transmitted diseases	People who have been **newly diagnosed with or have been treated for syphilis, gonorrhea, Chlamydia, or genital ulcers** in the preceding 12 months
NEW	People who have been on **hemodialysis** in the preceding 12 months (RISK FOR HCV ONLY)
Persons with hemophilia or related clotting disorders who have received human-derived clotting factor concentrates	Deleted

(Table 4.1) cont.....

1994 Guideline (All Ages)	2013 Guideline (All Ages)
Person who have been exposed in the preceding 12 months to known or suspected HIV-infected blood	Deleted
1994 Guideline (Pediatric)	**2013 Guideline (Pediatric)**
Children born to mothers with HIV infection or mothers who meet the behavioral or laboratory exclusionary criteria for adult donors (regardless of HIV status) should not be accepted as donors unless HIV infection can be definitely excluded in the child as follows: Children >18 months of age who are born to mothers with or at risk for HIV infection, who have not been breastfed within the last 12 months, and whose HIV Ab tests, physical exam, and review of medical records don not indicate evidence of HIV infection can be accepted as donors	A child who is ≤18 months of age and **born to a mother known to be infected with**, or at increased risk for HIV, HBV, or HCV infections
Children ≤18 months of age who are born to mothers with or at risk for HIV infection or who have been breastfed within the past 12 months should not be accepted as donors regardless of their HIV status	A child who has been **breastfed** within the preceding 12 months and the mother is known to be infected with, or at increased risk for HIV
1994 Guideline (Laboratory Findings)	**2013 Guideline (Laboratory Findings)**
Persons who cannot be tested for HIV infection because of refusal, inadequate blood samples (*e.g.* hemodilution that could result in a false negative test), or any other reasons	Any evidence of **hemodilution**
Persons with a repeatedly reactive screening assay for HIV-1 or HIV-2 Ab regardless of the result of supplemental assays.	
Persons whose history, physical exam, medical records, or autopsy reports reveal other evidence of HIV infection or high-risk behavior, such as a diagnosis of AIDS, unexplained weight loss, night sweats, blue or purple spots on the skin or mucous membranes typical of Kaposi's Sarcoma, unexplained lymphadenopathy lasting ≥ 1 month, unexplained temperature >100.5 F (38.6 C) for >10 days, unexplained persistent cough, MSM contact, sexually transmitted diseases, or needle tracks or other signs of parenteral drug abuse.	

Since the 2013 PHS guidelines were implemented, the percentage of donors that are labeled at increased risk has increased dramatically; 19.5% of donors from 2/1/2014-7/1/2014 were at increased risk as compared to 12.3% of donors from 2/1/2013-7/1/2013 [3]. Twenty-five of 58 U.S. OPOs now report > 25% of deceased donors are at increased risk as compared to only 5 OPOs with >25% increased risk donors previously [3]. The percentage of donors at increased risk is expected to continue to rise, especially given the current opioid epidemic in the U.S [3].

OPTN policy has always required OPOs to screen all organ donors with serology tests for HIV, HBV and HCV. After a well-publicized HIV/HCV transmission case in 2007, many OPOs began screening at least some donors with nucleic acid testing (NAT) in addition to serology to avoid transmissions of these viruses [4, 5], and NAT screening practices have expanded in the last decade [4, 6]. The PHS 2013 guidelines recommended NAT on a more regulated basis and OPTN updated policy in December, 2014 to state that all donors (regardless of increased risk status) be screened with HCV NAT and that increased risk donors be screened with HIV NAT [7]. NAT significantly decreases the amount of time between exposure to infection to detection by testing (window or eclipse period), therefore making the ability to detect more recent infection in higher risk donors much easier (Table **4.2**/Fig. **4.1**) [8 - 10].

Table 4.2. Window periods for serology *versus* NAT.

Virus	Serology	NAT
HIV	22 days	9 days
HBV	44 days	22 days
HCV	66 days	7 days

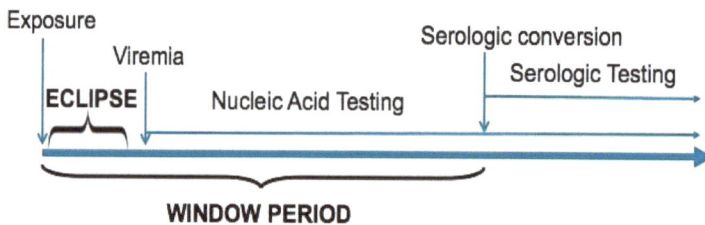

Fig. (4.1). Window periods for serology versus NAT. Medical Illustrations© 2018 Tim Phelps, MS, FAMI, Johns Hopkins University.

Even with the use of NAT, there have been transmissions reported [11]. The actual risk of transmission is estimated to be very low, even for the highest of risks, namely recent intravenous drug use. Estimations of risk from meta-analyses are shown in Table **4.3** [8, 9]. Exact risk of transmission is unknown. The risk of transmission is typically much lower than the risk of morbidity or mortality while awaiting an organ on the transplant list [12, 13]. It is important that transplant clinicians educate their transplant candidates about the risks and benefits of accepting organs from increased risk donors and a special informed consent prior to transplant is required by OPTN policy. Policy also states "...transplant programs must offer the recipients of organs from donors at increased risk for blood borne pathogens additional post-transplant testing for HIV, HCV, and/or

HBV (as appropriate based upon the recipient's pre-transplant status) and monitoring and/or therapy to treat or provide prophylaxis as appropriate to minimize the risk of infection in addition to routine post-transplant follow-up care [14]." Guidance on education of candidates can be found on the following websites: www.transplantmodels.com/IRD and https://optn.transplant.hrsa.gov/resources/guidance/understanding-hiv-hbv-hcv-risks-from-increased-risk-donors/.

Table 4.3. Risk of undetected HIV or HCV infection with Serology (ELISA) *versus* NAT [8, 9].

Risk per 10,000 Donors	HIV ELISA	HIV NAT	HCV ELISA	HCV NAT
Window Period	22 days	9 days	66 days	7 days
Men who have sex with men	8.3	3.4	36.0	3.8
IV Drug Users	12.9	5.3	350.0	37.8
Hemophiliacs	0.05	0.02	0.46	0.05
Commercial sex worker	2.9	1.2	107.8	11.5
Partner with the above	2.7	1.1	126.2	13.5
Blood product exposure	1.3	0.5	22.0	2.3
Incarceration	1.5	0.6	68.6	7.3

Although screening of recipients of increased risk donors is very important to be able to identify transmissions early, treat patients early, prevent complications of infections, and inform public health and policy, surveys have shown that, in practice, opportunities for screening are often missed [15]. Current recommendations are to screen all recipients of increased risk donor organs with HIV, HBV and HCV NAT between 1 and 3 months' post-transplant and with HBV serology at 1-year post-transplant [2]. It is critical that NAT is used to screen transplant recipients for these infections, especially in the case of HCV transmissions, since most patients never seroconvert [5, 11, 16].

Two recent related changes are worth noting. First, the HIV Organ Policy Equity Act made legal, under research protocols, the use of HIV-positive organs for HIV-positive recipients [17]; before this act, the use of HIV-positive organs was forbidden under any circumstances. Beyond the benefits of true HIV-positive donors, this also means that suspected false positive donors, which in the past were deemed as illegal as true positive donors, can now be used under HOPE protocols. A national, NIH-funded, multicenter study is underway to better understand the impact of HIV-positive donors (NCT02602262, U01AI134591, PI: Durand/Segev, Johns Hopkins University).

Another change is the drastic improvement of HCV treatment using direct-acting antivirals (DAAs). Most relevant to PHS increased risk donors is the prognosis, if a patient should acquire an undetected HCV infection, is much better than in the past, and the acquired HCV is likely curable.

Although donor HCV infection per se does not classify the donor as PHS increased risk, HCV viremic donors will inevitably transmit HCV to recipients without a preventive treatment protocol. As the number of patients with end-stage organ failure exceeds the donor supply, the use of HCV-viremic donor organs serves as a strategy to increase the donor pool. Among liver transplant recipients with chronic HCV infection, the use of HCV-viremic donor livers has been associated with comparable patient and graft survival to HCV-negative livers [18 - 20]. While several studies have demonstrated an increased mortality risk in HCV-positive patients receiving HCV-positive kidney transplants [21 - 23], receipt of an HCV-positive kidney appears to confer a survival advantage over remaining on dialysis [21].

In the current era of DAAs, which have shown efficacy in HCV-positive liver transplant recipients, the proportion of patients receiving HCV-positive donor livers for HCV-related end-stage liver disease has increased from 6.9% in 2010 to 16.9% in 2015 [24]. There are limited data regarding the treatment of HCV following non-hepatic transplant, though published reports suggest favorable cure rates with DAAs in this population [25]. DAAs have also been successfully utilized in the treatment of donor-derived hepatitis C infection in hepatic- and non-hepatic solid organ transplant recipients [26, 27].

The use of HCV-viremic donor organs in HCV-negative transplant recipients is not currently recommended, as this has previously been associated with mortality due to aggressive fibrosing cholestatic HCV [25]. Guidelines suggest that this may be considered in critically ill patients only if strict informed consent is obtained [28]. Two recent studies have shown promising success with HCV-viremic kidney transplants into HCV-negative recipients [29, 30]. On the other hand, HCV antibody positive, NAT negative (non-viremic) donors are at a very low risk of infection transmission [28].

CONSENT FOR PUBLICATION

Not applicable.

CONFLICT OF INTEREST

The author declares no conflict of interest, financial or otherwise.

ACKNOWLEDGEMENTS

Declared none.

REFERENCES

[1]   Guidelines for preventing transmission of human immunodeficiency virus through transplantation of human tissue and organs. MMWR Recomm Rep 1994; 43(RR-8): 1-17.
        [PMID: 8183226]

[2]   Seem DL, Lee I, Umscheid CA, Kuehnert MJ, Service USPH. PHS guideline for reducing human immunodeficiency virus, hepatitis B virus, and hepatitis C virus transmission through organ transplantation. Public Health Rep 2013; 128(4): 247-343.
        [http://dx.doi.org/10.1177/003335491312800403] [PMID: 23814319]

[3]   Kucirka LM, Bowring MG, Massie AB, Luo X, Nicholas LH, Segev DL. Landscape of deceased donors labeled increased risk for disease transmission under new guidelines. Am J Transplant 2015; 15(12): 3215-23.
        [http://dx.doi.org/10.1111/ajt.13356] [PMID: 26018059]

[4]   Theodoropoulos N, Jaramillo A, Ladner DP, Ison MG. Deceased organ donor screening for HIV, hepatitis B, and hepatitis C viruses: a survey of organ procurement organization practices. Am J Transplant 2013; 13(8): 2186-90.
        [http://dx.doi.org/10.1111/ajt.12260] [PMID: 23711196]

[5]   Ison MG, Llata E, Conover CS, *et al.* Transmission of human immunodeficiency virus and hepatitis C virus from an organ donor to four transplant recipients. Am J Transplant 2011; 11(6): 1218-25.
        [http://dx.doi.org/10.1111/j.1600-6143.2011.03597.x] [PMID: 21645254]

[6]   Kucirka LM, Alexander C, Namuyinga R, Hanrahan C, Montgomery RA, Segev DL. Viral nucleic acid testing (NAT) and OPO-level disposition of high-risk donor organs. Am J Transplant 2009; 9(3): 620-8.
        [http://dx.doi.org/10.1111/j.1600-6143.2008.02522.x] [PMID: 19191766]

[7]   OPTN Policy 2.0 Deceased Donor Organ Procurement. http://optntransplanthrsagov/media/1200/optn_policiespdf#nameddest=Policy_02 [Internet] 2016 January 4; Available from: http://optn.transplant.hrsa.gov/ContentDocuments/OPTN_Policies.pdf#nameddest=Policy_02

[8]   Kucirka LM, Sarathy H, Govindan P, *et al.* Risk of window period hepatitis-C infection in high infectious risk donors: systematic review and meta-analysis. Am J Transplant 2011; 11(6): 1188-200.
        [http://dx.doi.org/10.1111/j.1600-6143.2011.03460.x] [PMID: 21401874]

[9]   Kucirka LM, Sarathy H, Govindan P, *et al.* Risk of window period HIV infection in high infectious risk donors: systematic review and meta-analysis. Am J Transplant 2011; 11(6): 1176-87.
        [http://dx.doi.org/10.1111/j.1600-6143.2010.03329.x] [PMID: 21366859]

[10]   Theodoropoulos N, Ison MG, Jaramillo A. Screening deceased organ donors for infectious disease: optimization of testing. ASHI Quarterly 2012; 36(3): 18-26.

[11]   Suryaprasad A, Basavaraju SV, Hocevar SN, *et al.* Organ Transplantation Hepatitis C Investigation Team. Transmission of hepatitis C virus from organ donors despite nucleic acid test screening. Am J Transplant 2015; 15(7): 1827-35.
        [http://dx.doi.org/10.1111/ajt.13283] [PMID: 25943299]

[12]   Chow EK, Massie AB, Muzaale AD, *et al.* Identifying appropriate recipients for CDC infectious risk donor kidneys. Am J Transplant 2013; 13(5): 1227-34.
        [http://dx.doi.org/10.1111/ajt.12206] [PMID: 23621162]

[13]   Bowring MG, Holscher CM, Zhou S, *et al.* Turn down for what? Patient outcomes associated with declining increased infectious risk kidneys. Am J Transplant 2018; 18(3): 617-24.
        [http://dx.doi.org/10.1111/ajt.14577] [PMID: 29116674]

[14]   OPTN Policy 15. Identification of Transmissible Diseases. http://optntransplanthrsagov/ ContentDocuments/OPTN_Policiespdf#nameddest=Policy_02 [Internet] 2015 April 27; Available from: http://optn.transplant.hrsa.gov/ContentDocuments/OPTN_Policies.pdf#nameddest=Policy_02

[15]   Theodoropoulos N, Ladner DP, Ison MG. Screening recipients of increased-risk donor organs: a survey of transplant infectious diseases physician practices. Transpl Infect Dis 2013; 15(5): 545-9. [PMID: 23901896]

[16]   Ison MG. Nucleic acid testing of organ donors: is the glass half empty or half full? Am J Transplant 2015; 15(7): 1743-5. [http://dx.doi.org/10.1111/ajt.13289] [PMID: 25943975]

[17]   Boyarsky BJ, Segev DL. From bench to bill: how a transplant nuance became 1 of only 57 laws passed in 2013. Ann Surg 2016; 263(3): 430-3. [http://dx.doi.org/10.1097/SLA.0000000000001352] [PMID: 26575282]

[18]   Northup PG, Argo CK, Nguyen DT, *et al.* Liver allografts from hepatitis C positive donors can offer good outcomes in hepatitis C positive recipients: a US National Transplant Registry analysis. Transpl Int 2010; 23(10): 1038-44. [http://dx.doi.org/10.1111/j.1432-2277.2010.01092.x] [PMID: 20444239]

[19]   Álvaro E, Abradelo M, Fuertes A, *et al.* Liver transplantation from anti-hepatitis C virus-positive donors: our experience. Transplant Proc 2012; 44(6): 1475-8. [http://dx.doi.org/10.1016/j.transproceed.2012.05.012] [PMID: 22841188]

[20]   Marroquin CE, Marino G, Kuo PC, *et al.* Transplantation of hepatitis C-positive livers in hepatitis C-positive patients is equivalent to transplanting hepatitis C-negative livers. Liver Transpl 2001; 7(9): 762-8. [http://dx.doi.org/10.1053/jlts.2001.27088] [PMID: 11552208]

[21]   Abbott KC, Bucci JR, Matsumoto CS, *et al.* Hepatitis C and renal transplantation in the era of modern immunosuppression. J Am Soc Nephrol 2003; 14(11): 2908-18. [http://dx.doi.org/10.1097/01.ASN.0000090743.43034.72] [PMID: 14569101]

[22]   Bucci JR, Matsumoto CS, Swanson SJ, *et al.* Donor hepatitis C seropositivity: clinical correlates and effect on early graft and patient survival in adult cadaveric kidney transplantation. J Am Soc Nephrol 2002; 13(12): 2974-82. [http://dx.doi.org/10.1097/01.ASN.0000034944.90425.75] [PMID: 12444217]

[23]   Maluf DG, Archer KJ, Villamil F, Stravitz RT, Mas V. Hepatitis C virus recurrence after liver transplantation: biomarkers of disease and fibrosis progression. Expert Rev Gastroenterol Hepatol 2010; 4(4): 445-58. [http://dx.doi.org/10.1586/egh.10.39] [PMID: 20678018]

[24]   Bowring MG, Kucirka LM, Massie AB, *et al.* Changes in utilization and discard of hepatitis C-infected donor livers in the recent era. Am J Transplant 2017; 17(2): 519-27. [http://dx.doi.org/10.1111/ajt.13976] [PMID: 27456927]

[25]   Belga S, Doucette KE. Hepatitis C in non-hepatic solid organ transplant candidates and recipients: A new horizon. World J Gastroenterol 2016; 22(4): 1650-63. [http://dx.doi.org/10.3748/wjg.v22.i4.1650] [PMID: 26819530]

[26]   Shah AP, Cameron A, Singh P, Frank AM, Fenkel JM. Successful treatment of donor-derived hepatitis C viral infection in three transplant recipients from a donor at increased risk for bloodborne pathogens. Transpl Infect Dis 2017; 19(2) [http://dx.doi.org/10.1111/tid.12660] [PMID: 28060446]

[27]   Theodoropoulos N, Whitson BA, Martin SI, Pouch S, Pope-Harman A. Successful treatment of donor-derived hepatitis C infection in a lung transplant recipient. Transpl Infect Dis 2017; 19(2) [http://dx.doi.org/10.1111/tid.12659] [PMID: 28060441]

[28]   Levitsky J, Doucette K. AST Infectious Diseases Community of Practice. Viral hepatitis in solid organ

transplantation. Am J Transplant 2013; 13 (Suppl. 4): 147-68.
[http://dx.doi.org/10.1111/ajt.12108] [PMID: 23465008]

[29]   Durand CM, Bowring MG, Brown DM, *et al.* Direct-acting antiviral prophylaxis in kidney transplantation from hepatitis c virus-infected donors to noninfected recipients: an open-label nonrandomized trial. Ann Intern Med 2018; 168(8): 533-40. Epub ahead of print
[http://dx.doi.org/10.7326/M17-2871] [PMID: 29507971]

[30]   Goldberg DS, Abt PL, Blumberg EA, *et al.* Trial of transplantation of HCV-infected kidneys into uninfected recipients. N Engl J Med 2017; 376(24): 2394-5.
[http://dx.doi.org/10.1056/NEJMc1705221] [PMID: 28459186]

CHAPTER 5

Management of the Multi-Organ Donor and Logistic Considerations

Sharon Weeks[*], **Shane Ottmann** and **Andrew Cameron**

Johns Hopkins University School of Medicine, Baltimore, MD, USA

Abstract: This chapter examines the effect of brain death physiology on potentially recoverable organs and provides specific management recommendations for the care of the multi-organ donor. We also review the logistic considerations important for successful procurement. The goal of these aims is to optimize function and maximize recovery of life-saving organs.

Keywords: Multi-Organ Donor, Organ Procurement, Transplant Logistic Considerations.

INTRODUCTION

Once a potential organ donor is identified, it is important to actively manage physiologic changes that take place after brain death as many changes have adverse effects on organ suitability and function. Particularly as absolute and relative contraindications to organ donation have declined in recent years, the management of potential donor organs has become more complex (Table **5.1**). Potential donors are also now more likely to be patients at the extremes of age or be marginal or extended criteria donors [1 - 3]. Additionally, patients with previously absolute contraindications such as HIV infection are now potential organ donors because of policy changes to implement the HIV Organ Policy Equity Act [4]. These changes in policy present new challenges in the management of the potential multi-organ donor, but support the ultimate goal of maximizing the number of transplantable organs.

Brainstem death leads to inevitable dysautonomia with progressive cardiovascular dysfunction and pulmonary deterioration. Loss of thermal regulation and the hypothalamopituitary neuroendocrine axis results in temperature dysregulation, declining metabolism, loss of volume homeostasis, and hormone abnormalities.

---

[*] **Corresponding author Sharon Weeks:** Johns Hopkins University School of Medicine, Baltimore, MD, USA; Tel: 410-502-5198; Fax: 410-510-1514; Email: sweeks@jhmi.edu

Targeted and active management of the potential donor from brain death to organ procurement requires a shift in management from cerebral protection toward preserving organ perfusion and function [5]. Standardizing donor management reduces the rate of family refusal of donation, decreases the number of donors lost to circulatory collapse, and transforms some unacceptable donors to acceptable [6]. The Papworth program in Great Britain demonstrated that hemodynamic management and hormonal therapy converted to successful donors 85% of brain patients who, at initial assessment, fell outside the acceptance guidelines [7]. The goal of active management of potential donors is thus to optimize function for the maximum number of organs.

Table 5.1. Absolute contraindications to organ donation.

Severe trauma – does not preclude donation of unaffected organs
Malignancy outside the central nervous system
Active infections

DONOR MANAGEMENT

Cardiovascular Dysfunction

Managing the cardiovascular changes in the potential donor following brain death is important to maintain functionality of transplantable organs. The rostral-caudal progression of brainstem ischemia that results in brain death is often characterized by autonomic surge after medullary ischemia to maintain cerebral perfusion pressures [8]. This "catecholamine storm" is not clinically apparent in all patients, but can present with increased cardiac output, heart rate and systemic vascular resistance. There may also be signs of myocardial ischemia, conduction abnormalities, and arrhythmias [9]. This period is short, lasting on average 1.2 hours with a range of 30 minutes to 6 hours in one study [10], and usually self-resolving. While some have advocated treatment of autonomic storm to improve cardiac graft function, a goal of organ preservation over cerebral protection is problematic in this clinical scenario, which typically precedes brain death pronouncement [8].

Progression of ischemia to the spinal cord level and resulting brain death are characterized by progressive loss of sympathetic tone and peripheral vasodilation, leading to systemic hypoperfusion, ischemia, and eventual cardiovascular collapse. Intrinsic cardiac function is also reduced, secondary to catecholamine cardiotoxicity or myocardial demand ischemia; histologic exam of cardiac tissue after autonomic storm reveals widespread ischemia and necrosis [11 - 13]. Echocardiography, preferably transesophageal, has been advocated to rule out major structural abnormalities and to measure left ventricular ejection fraction (LVEF) [14]. Transient wall motion abnormalities can be common and may resolve with adequate hemodynamic management [9].

Central venous access to monitor pressures accurately is necessary for proper donor management [9]. For potential lung donors, central venous pressure (CVP) of less than 8 mm Hg is recommended; higher pressures result in increased alveolar to arterial oxygen gradients [15]. However, for optimal perfusion of the abdominal organs, CVP is ideally maintained at 10-12 mm Hg. Consequently, in the multi-organ donor, a CVP of 8-10 has been proposed as a reasonable compromise [16]. Failure to achieve this goal should prompt aggressive fluid resuscitation [17]. Mean arterial pressure (MAP) less than 60-65 mm Hg despite resuscitation should prompt investigation for other causes of hypotension, such as hemorrhage (either from previous acute bleed or secondary to coagulopathy) or hypovolemia from unaddressed diabetes insipidus. The use of catecholamines in the donor is associated with impaired gas exchange and thus should be minimized whenever possible [18], but is used to treat hypotension in the non-anemic, fluid replete patient. Dopamine is the first line vasopressor for potential donors; it improves both immediate and long-term renal graft function and is associated with faster alveolar fluid clearance [19, 20]. Vasopressin decreases inotropic needs, treats diabetes insipidus, and aids in the correction of neurogenic hypotension *via* anti-inflammatory mechanisms [21 - 23].

Goals of fluid resuscitation include MAP ≥ 60, urinary output ≥ 1 cc/kg/hr, LVEF ≥ 45% and minimal vasoactive agents (dopamine ≤ 10 μg/kg/min). Insertion of a pulmonary artery catheter may be necessary if ejection fraction is less than 40% or if hemodynamic instability persists after volume resuscitation [8, 9]. Goals with such monitoring include pulmonary capillary wedge pressure (PCWP) 6-10 mmHg, cardiac index > 2.4 L/min m^2 and systemic vascular resistance 800-1200 dynes s cm^{-5} [8, 24]. Norepinephrine is used for hemodynamic instability unresponsive to fluid resuscitation and dopamine administration. Persistently refractory hypotension may be treated with hormonal therapy as a last resort.

Tension exists between the competing interests of renal and pulmonary grafts that complicate fluid management in the multiorgan donor. Kidney function is improved with maintenance of adequate urine output related to expanded intravascular volume while lung function is enhanced by diminished intravascular volume to prevent extravascular lung water accumulation [8]. Early assessment of whether the donor is a potential lung donor can help guide management. Optimal fluid replacement is debated, but should consist of colloid for intravascular expansion, blood to maintain hematocrit of 30%, and crystalloid with electrolytes to replace urinary losses. Addition of dextrose is important to maintain hepatic stores.

Pulmonary Deterioration

The lungs may suffer injury for multiple reasons that prevent suitability for transplantation: direct trauma, resuscitation maneuvers, neurogenic edema, aspiration, or ventilator associated trauma or pneumonia. The lungs are the organ most often deemed medically unsuitable, with a recovery rate from deceased donors of 23% [25]. Physiologically, the catecholamine surge seen in brain dead patients can have profound effects on pulmonary function. Increased systemic vascular resistance leads to left ventricular dysfunction, creating a hydrostatic gradient that precipitates pulmonary edema. Vasoconstriction increases venous return, resulting in increased right heart pressures and pulmonary blood flow. In combination with the failure of capillary-alveolar membrane integrity following brain death, this higher pulmonary capillary pressure and blood flow leads to pulmonary edema [8, 11, 26]. The neurogenic hypotension that follows sympathetic storm activates a systemic inflammatory syndrome, which leads to further trauma to the lungs from neutrophil infiltration and migration into the pulmonary interstitial and alveolar space. Finally, pulmonary dysfunction in the brain dead donor is often associated with aspiration, pneumonia, contusion, and ventilator-associated injury [11].

Practically speaking, there are several measures to maximize pulmonary suitability of a potential organ donor. A goal of SaO2 > 95% should be maintained. Some advocate for a lung protective ventilator strategy of tidal volumes of 6-8 ml/kg, as employed in ARDS, to prevent barotrauma [26], while others, including the San Antonio Lung Transplant protocol, recommend more traditional ventilator settings of 10-12 ml/kg [5, 27]. Peak inspiratory pressures less than 30 cm H_2O and FiO2 of less than 40% to prevent oxygen toxicity are recommended. Recruitment maneuvers and PEEP of 5-10 cm H_2O combat and prevent atelectasis. Elevation of the head of bed and adequate endotracheal cuff pressures to 25 cm H_2O help prevent aspiration. Pulmonary toilet with physiotherapy and frequent endotracheal suctioning increases rates of lung procurement and organ quality [27]. Avoiding overventilation and resultant respiratory alkalosis will prevent a metabolic acidosis that contributes to further systemic hypoperfusion. Bronchoscopy is routinely performed on potential lung donors to assess for airway damage and signs of infection [5, 9, 11, 26]. Animal and *ex vivo* studies demonstrated increased alveolar fluid clearance with β_2-adrenergic stimulation, though a randomized controlled trial of over 500 potential donors given high dose aerosolized albuterol showed increased tachycardia without improvement in donor oxygenation or lung utilization [28].

Though kidney graft function is improved with aggressive fluid resuscitation, hypervolemia will compound right ventricular dysfunction with potentially deleterious effects on the lungs. Thus, in potential thoracic donors, normovolemia should be the goal. Colloid may be the preferred fluid to minimize accumulation of pulmonary edema and deterioration in gas exchange; crystalloid is minimized and diuretics are used as necessary to achieve neutral or negative fluid balance [27]. High-dose methylprednisolone after brain death was associated with reduced extravascular lung water, improved oxygenation and increased lung donor utilization, likely by limiting cytokine-mediated cellular injury [21, 29]. Protocol based strategies for potential lungs donors have repeatedly demonstrated increased procurement rates [21, 27].

Endocrine Derangements

Disruption of the hypothalamopituitary neuroendocrine axis and the effect on a donor's endocrine system remain an area of active inquiry. Anterior pituitary function is typically preserved, but deficiencies in T3, T4, ACTH, TSH and growth hormone have been described in both animal and human studies. The clinical relevance of these deficiencies remains an open question as conflicting evidence in organ donors have been reported. Animal studies have demonstrated improved hemodynamics and organ function after brain death with supplementation with triiodothyronine, insulin, and cortisol [30, 31]. Similarly, human studies in organ donors have demonstrated decreased need for vasoactive support and increased rates of transplantable organs when donors are given exogenous hormones (methylprednisolone, vasopressin and triiodothyronine) [32 - 34]. However, other studies show aggressive volume replacement was sufficient to achieve similarly effective hemodynamic outcomes and that no correlation existed between hormonal levels and hemodynamics after brain death [35, 36]. Systematic reviews advocate against routine use of thyroid hormone replacement for stable donors but report a possible role as a rescue therapy in potential donors with persistent hemodynamic instability [37, 38]. A randomized controlled trial of potential cardiac donors did not demonstrate improved cardiovascular function or graft yield with use of triiodothyronine and methylprednisolone [39]. Despite this conflict in the literature, many published donor management programs, which show excellent results in donor utilization, include hormonal therapy as part of their protocols. Both the Papworth program and Crystal City Consensus, for example, use bolus steroids, insulin and glucose, vasopressin and thyroid hormones as rescue therapy for hemodynamically unsuitable patients [5, 7]. UNOS recommends combined hormone therapy of triiodothyronine, vasopressin, and methylprednisone for all cardiothoracic donors [40]. Some advocate for consideration of triple therapy in all donors on the basis of large retrospective cohort study showing decreased vasoactive support and increased recovery of heart, liver, and kidney grafts [9, 32].

While anterior pituitary function remains an open question, there appears to be clear loss of posterior pituitary function, which manifests as diabetes insipidus in up to 80% of potential donors [16]. Undetectable levels of ADH were noted in 75% of donors and were associated with hemodynamic instability and compromised function of transplanted organs [9]. The resulting diuresis exacerbates the intravascular hypovolemia seen after brain death and combats attempts at adequate fluid resuscitation. It also results in electrolyte imbalances, primarily hypernatremia, which is concerning for hepatic grafts as early studies reported association with significant hepatic graft dysfunction [41, 42]. More recent data question whether severe hypernatremia causes primary nonfunction in the transplanted liver and report similar outcomes of early liver function and one year risk of failure between groups with varying degrees of hypernatremia [43]. Nevertheless, sodium levels are typically corrected in donor management protocols. Treatment of diabetes insipidus typically consists of volume replacement to combat fluid losses, vasopressin supplementation for antidiuretic effect, as well as identification and treatment of other causes of polyuria, including previous osmotic therapy for increased intracranial pressure, hyperglycemia or diuretic agents [44].

Temperature Regulation

Destruction of the hypothalamic thermoregulatory center renders the brain dead patient essentially poikilothermic, predisposing to arrhythmias and impairing oxygen delivery. In potential donors, hypothermia is associated with declining renal function, pancreatitis, cold-induced diuresis, and coagulopathies. Active steps to prevent hypothermia and maintain normothermia should be taken including warming and humidifying ventilator gases, warming intravenous fluids, and using external warming devices such as convective warm air blankets.

LOGISTIC CONSIDERATIONS

Organizational Considerations

As the number of brain dead individuals is limited and represents only 1% of all deaths [45], the conversion of potential donors to actual organ donors is critical to maximize organ transplantation [46]. Most countries with active transplantation programs have an organizational model to facilitate the logistics of this complex process. These include the in-hospital "Spanish model" and the extra-hospital organ procurement organizations (OPOs) seen the United States. Regardless of structure, these organizations work to increase efficiency and efficacy in donor detection (identification and screening), donor maintenance, brain death diagnosis, consent, organ allocation, and coordination of recovery surgery with an effort to balance family, donor, and recipient needs. ***The primary goal of every organization is to maximize the greatest number of transplants from each potential donor while avoiding damage to quality organs in attempts to rescue and place marginal organs.*** Logistic orchestration to achieve this goal includes timely allocation of organs, balancing the needs of multiple surgical teams for procurement timing, and respecting constraints arising from the local hospital, family or donor needs.

The Spanish model for organ donation and transplantation has long been regarded as a success story in increasing organ donation rates on a country-wide level. The National Organization of Transplants (ONT, Organización Nacional de Trasplantes) was started in September 1989 under the auspices of the Department of Health to create an integrated transplant organization program based on a network of well-trained transplant coordinators [47]. Local coordinators, who are based in hospitals and are typically intensivists who devote part time work to organ transplantation, work in concert with counterparts at the regional and national level [48, 49]. Coordinators are trained through an extensive program [50] on identification of donors, techniques in diagnosing brain death, clinical management and maintenance of the donor, psychological approaches to the grieving family, and consent procedures, as well as the ethics and law surrounding transplantation [47]. In addition to this foundation at the local level, the Spanish model involves a comprehensive national program of education, communication, public relations, hospital reimbursement and quality improvement [51]. As a result of this coordinated effort, Spain boasted 40.2 donors per million population in 2015, the world's highest rate of organ donation (Fig. **5.1**) [52].

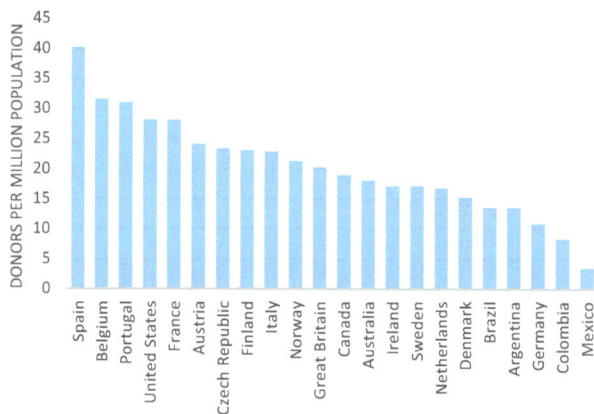

Fig. (5.1). Global annual rates of organ donation from actual deceased donors. Medical Illustrations© 2018 Tim Phelps, MS, FAMI, Johns Hopkins University.

In the United States, the National Organ Transplant Act of 1984 established Organ Procurement Organizations (OPOs) as charitable non-profit organizations responsible for promoting organ donation, identifying potential organ donors, and for recovering and distributing organs for transplantation. Each OPO serves a defined "donation service area" (DSA) and has agreements in place with each hospital within that geographic area to coordinate donation, recovery, and transplant. A donor referral to the OPO, as mandated by law for hospital deaths or imminent deaths, prompts initiation of a process to evaluate the potential organ donor and recover and subsequently transplant as many organs as possible. Only hospitals that report deaths or potential deaths in a timely fashion to the local OPO are considered by the Centers for Medicare & Medicaid Services (CMS) to have met "conditions of participation," which determines eligibility to receive Medicare benefits [53]. The Joint Commission also requires that hospitals maintain a written agreement with an OPO for the purposes of organ and tissue donation and procurement. To this end, the local OPO identifies and medically evaluates potential organ donors and coordinates the recovery, transportation, and placement of the donated organ.

Logistics of Organ Recovery

Organ procurement is the culmination of efforts by the coordinating team following the allocation (*i.e.* placement) of each suitable organ for transplantation and arrangement of recipient operating room schedules as well as recovery team travel arrangements. Organ allocation is driven by organ specific algorithms that are continually assessed and updated as needed to address the Final Rule, which replaced locally driven allocation with a single national distribution pool and prioritized medical urgency over waitlist time [54, 55]. Once allocation of transplantable organs is complete, the coordinator arranges for operating room time at the donor hospital, which typically also provides anesthesia, nursing support, and surgical technologists. This time must also be coordinated with the procurement surgical teams as they ready transplant recipients, particularly for time sensitive cardiac, pulmonary, and hepatic grafts. Ideally, delays to this process are minimal to prevent disruption of donor care and compromise of organs. However, donor stability, constraints placed by the family of the donor, or logistical issues at recipient transplant centers may all play a role in procurement timing. The coordinator and surgical teams must also work together to ensure that all needed surgical instruments, perfusion solutions and materials, and medications needed for the procurement will be available.

Surgical teams from recipient hospitals usually recover the organs for their recipients. Cardiothoracic teams almost always perform their own organ retrievals. However, the presence of one abdominal team helps streamline the process; local teams often procure kidneys for other transplant centers [56]. Communication and professionalism between surgical teams is critical. It is necessary to discuss the details of technique and sequence of events prior to beginning a procurement. Typically, the order of multiple organ procurement gives priority to heart and lungs, then liver, pancreas and small bowel, then kidneys, vascular grafts, and tissues. The coordinator documents the procurement process, prepares the donor for tissue banking, and attends to care of the donor after donation. They are also responsible for preserving, labeling, packaging and transporting organs.

CONCLUSION

The time from identification of a potential organ donor to transplantation of suitable organs is a critical period to achieve the goal of maximizing the greatest number of transplanted organs of the highest function from each potential donor. The complex process must be actively managed, both through medical care of the potential donor and in coordinating the complex logistics of allocation, recovery of organs, and eventual transplantation surgeries (Fig. **5.2**). Importantly, much of this work is performed outside active transplant centers, by local donor hospitals and the local OPO (or other organizational system outside the US). Effective management of this process increases donor rates and organ utilization, maximizes benefit to recipients, and allows the donor's loved ones to realize some benefit and closure at a difficult time.

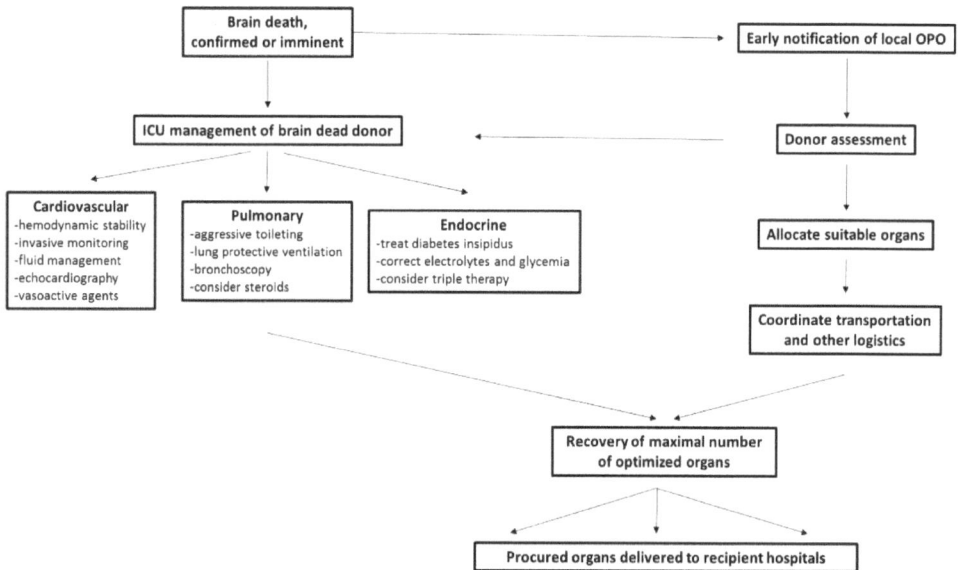

Fig. (5.2). Algorithm for management of the potential multi-organ donor. Medical Illustrations© 2018 Tim Phelps, MS, FAMI, Johns Hopkins University.

CONSENT FOR PUBLICATION

Not applicable.

CONFLICT OF INTEREST

The author declares no conflict of interest, financial or otherwise.

ACKNOWLEDGEMENTS

Declared none.

REFERENCES

[1]   Tullius SG, Volk HD, Neuhaus P. Transplantation of organs from marginal donors. Transplantation 2001; 72(8): 1341-9.
[http://dx.doi.org/10.1097/00007890-200110270-00001]

[2]   Audard V, Matignon M, Dahan K, Lang P, Grimbert P. Renal transplantation from extended criteria cadaveric donors: Problems and perspectives overview. Transpl Int 2008; 21(1): 11-7.

[3]   Tuttle-Newhall JE, Collins BH, Kuo PC, Schoeder R. Organ donation and treatment of the multi-organ donor. Curr Probl Surg 2003; 40(5): 266-310.
[http://dx.doi.org/10.1067/msg.2003.120005]

[4]   Health Resources and Services Administration (HRSA), Department of Health and Human Services (HHS). Organ procurement and transplantation: implementation of the HIV Organ Policy Equity Act. Final rule. Fed Regist 2015; 80(89): 26464-7.

[5]   Rosengard BR, Feng S, Alfrey EJ, *et al.* Report of the crystal city meeting to maximize the use of organs recovered from the cadaver donor. Am J Transplant 2002; 2(8): 701-11.
[http://dx.doi.org/10.1034/j.1600-6143.2002.20804.x]

[6]   Salim A, Martin M, Brown C, Rhee P, Demetriades D, Belzberg H. The effect of a protocol of aggressive donor management: Implications for the national organ donor shortage. J Trauma 2006; 61(2): 429-433-435.

[7]   Wheeldon D, Potter C, Oduro A, Wallwork J, Large S. Transforming the "unacceptable" donor: outcomes from the adoption of a standardized donor management technique. J Heart Lung Transplant 1995; 14(4): 734-42.

[8]   Wood KE, McCartney J. Management of the potential organ donor. Transplant Rev (Orlando) 2007; 21: 204-18.
[http://dx.doi.org/10.1016/j.trre.2007.07.007]

[9]   Mascia L, Mastromauro I, Viberti S, Vincenzi M, Zanello M. Management to optimize organ procurement in brain dead donors. Minerva Anestesiol 2009; 75: 125-33.

[10]   Audibert G, Charpentier C, Seguin-Devaux C, Charretier P-A, Grégoire H, Devaux Y, *et al.* Improvement of donor myocardial function after treatment of autonomic storm during brain death. Transplantation 2006; 82(8): 1031-6.
[http://dx.doi.org/10.1097/01.tp.0000235825.97538.d5]

[11]   Bugge JF. Brain death and its implications for management of the potential organ donor. Acta Anaesthesiol Scand 2009; 53(10): 1239-50.
[http://dx.doi.org/10.1111/j.1399-6576.2009.02064.x]

[12]   Li J, Konstantinov IE, Cai S, Shimizu M, Redington AN. Systemic and myocardial oxygen transport responses to brain death in pigs. Transplant Proc 2007; 39(1): 21-6.

[http://dx.doi.org/10.1016/j.transproceed.2006.10.201]

[13]   Wilhelm MJ, Pratschke J. Laskowski I a, Paz DM, Tilney NL. Brain death and its impact on the donor heart-lessons from animal models. J Heart Lung Transplant 2000; 19(5): 414-8.
[http://dx.doi.org/10.1016/S1053-2498(00)00073-5]

[14]   Cipolla J, Stawicki S, Spatz D. Hemodynamic monitoring of organ donors: A novel use of the esophageal echo-Doppler probe. Am Surg 2006; 72(6): 500-4.

[15]   Potter C, Wheeldon D, Wallwork J. Functional assessment and management of heart donors: a rationale for characterization and a guide to therapy. J Hear Lung Transplant1 1995; 14: 59-65.

[16]   Brockmann JG, Vaidya A, Reddy S, Friend PJ. Retrieval of abdominal organs for transplantation. Br J Surg 2006; 93: 133-46.
[http://dx.doi.org/10.1002/bjs.5228]

[17]   Powner DJ, Darby J. Management of variations in blood pressure during care of organ donors. Prog Transplant (Aliso Viejo, Calif)2 2000; 10: 25-30.

[18]   Mukadam ME, Harrington DK, Wilson IC, *et al.* Does donor catecholamine administration affect early lung function after transplantation? J Thorac Cardiovasc Surg 2005; 130(3): 926-7.
[http://dx.doi.org/10.1016/j.jtcvs.2005.02.007]

[19]   Schnuelle P, Berger S, de Boer J, Persijn G, van der Woude FJ. Effects of catecholamine application to brain-dead donors on graft survival in solid organ transplantation. Transplantation 2001; 72(3): 455-63.
[http://dx.doi.org/10.1097/00007890-200108150-00017]

[20]   Ware L, Fang X, Wany Y, Sakuma T, Hall T, Matthay M. Lung edema clearance: 20 years of progress. J Appl Physiol 2002; 93: 1869-74.
[http://dx.doi.org/10.1152/japplphysiol.00252.2002]

[21]   Venkateswaran RV. Early donor management increases the retrieval rate of lungs for transplantation. Ann Thorac Surg 2008; 85(1): 278-86.
[http://dx.doi.org/10.1016/j.athoracsur.2007.07.092]

[22]   Pennefather S, Bullock R, Mantle D, Dark J. Use of low dose arginine vasopressin to support brain-dead organ donors. Transplantation 1995; 59: 5-62.
[http://dx.doi.org/10.1097/00007890-199501150-00011]

[23]   Rostron AJ, Avlonitis VS, Cork DMW, Grenade DS, Kirby JA, Dark JH. Hemodynamic resuscitation with arginine vasopressin reduces lung injury after brain death in the transplant donor. Transplantation 2008; 85(4): 597-606.
[http://dx.doi.org/10.1097/TP.0b013e31816398dd]

[24]   Smith M. Physiologic changes during brain stem death: lessons for management of the organ donor. J Hear Lung Transpl 2004; 23(9 Suppl): S217-22.

[25]   OPTN. 2016 Annual Report of the US Organ Procurement and Transplantation Network and the Scientific Registry of Transplant Recipients Department of Health and Human Services Administration, Healthcare Systems Bureau, Division of Transplantation, Rockville, MD; United Network for Organ Sharing, Richmond, VA. Ann Arbor, MI: University Renal Research and Education Association 2016.

[26]   Van Raemdonck D, Neyrinck A, Verleden GM, *et al.* Lung Donor Selection and Management. Proc Am Thorac Soc 2009; 6: 28-38.
[http://dx.doi.org/10.1513/pats.200808-098GO]

[27]   Angel LF, Levine DJ, Restrepo MI, *et al.* Impact of a lung transplantation donor-management protocol on lung donation and recipient outcomes. Am J Respir Crit Care Med 2006; 174(6): 710-6.
[http://dx.doi.org/10.1164/rccm.200603-432OC]

[28]   Ware LB, Landeck M, Koyama T, *et al.* A Randomized Trial of the Effects of Nebulized Albuterol on

Pulmonary Edema in Brain Dead Organ Donors. Am J Transplant 2014; 14(3): 621-8.
[http://dx.doi.org/10.1111/ajt.12564]

[29]   Follette D, Rudich S, Babcock W. Improved oxygenation and increased lung donor recovery with high-dose steroid administration after brain death. J Heart Lung Transplant 1998; 17(4): 423-9.

[30]   Cooper D, Novitzky D, Wicomb W. Hormonal therapy in the brain-dead experimental animal. Transpl Proc1 1988; 20: 50-4.

[31]   Wicomb W, Cooper D, Novitzky D. Impairment of renal slice function following brain death, with reversibility of injury by hormonal therapy. Transplantation 1986; 41: 29-33.
[http://dx.doi.org/10.1097/00007890-198601000-00005]

[32]   Rosendale JD, Kauffman HM, McBride M, *et al.* Aggressive pharmacologic donor management results in more transplanted organs. Transplantation 2003; 75(4): 482-7.
[http://dx.doi.org/10.1097/01.TP.0000045683.85282.93]

[33]   Novitzky D, Cooper D. Results of hormonal therapy in human brain-dead potential organ donors. Transplant Proc 1988; 20: 59-62.

[34]   Novitzky D, Mi Z, Sun Q, Collins JF, Cooper DKC. Thyroid hormone therapy in the management of 63,593 brain-dead organ donors: a retrospective analysis. Transplantation 2014; 98(10): 1119-27.
[http://dx.doi.org/10.1097/TP.0000000000000187]

[35]   Goarin J-P, Cohen S, Riou B, *et al.* The Effects of Triiodothyronine on Hemodynamic Status and Cardiac Function in Potential Heart Donors. Anesth Analg 1996; 83: 41-7.
[http://dx.doi.org/10.1213/00000539-199607000-00008]

[36]   Powner D, Hendrich A, Lagler R, Ng R, Madden R. Hormonal changes in brain dead patients. Crit Care Med 1990; 18: 702-8.
[http://dx.doi.org/10.1097/00003246-199007000-00004]

[37]   Powner DJ, Hernandez M. A review of thyroid hormone administration during adult donor care. Prog Transplant 2005; 15(3): 202-7.
[http://dx.doi.org/10.1177/152692480501500302]

[38]   Macdonald PS, Aneman A, Bhonagiri D, *et al.* A systematic review and meta-analysis of clinical trials of thyroid hormone administration to brain dead potential organ donors. Crit Care Med 2012; 40(5): 1635-44.
[http://dx.doi.org/10.1097/CCM.0b013e3182416ee7]

[39]   Venkateswaran RV, Steeds RP, Quinn DW, *et al.* The haemodynamic effects of adjunctive hormone therapy in potential heart donors: A prospective randomized double-blind factorially designed controlled trial. Eur Heart J 2009; 30(14): 1771-80.
[http://dx.doi.org/10.1093/eurheartj/ehp086]

[40]   United Network for Organ Sharing (UNOS). Critical Pathway for the Organ Donor [cited: 31 July 2017] http://www.unos.org

[41]   Markmann J, Markmann J, Markmann D, *et al.* Preoperative factors associated with outcome and their impact on resource use in 1148 consecutive primary liver transplants. Transplantation 2001; 72(6): 1113-22.
[http://dx.doi.org/10.1097/00007890-200109270-00023]

[42]   Totsuka E, Dodson F. Influence of high donor serum sodium levels on early postoperative graft function in human liver transplantation: effect of correction of donor hypernatremia. Liver Transpl 1999; 5(5): 421-8.
[http://dx.doi.org/10.1002/lt.500050510]

[43]   Mangus RS, Fridell JA, Vianna RM, *et al.* Severe Hypernatremia in Deceased Liver Donors Does Not Impact Early Transplant Outcome. Clin Transplational Res 2010; 90: 438-43.

[44]   Dictus C, Vienenkoetter B, Esmaeilzadeh M, Unterberg A, Ahmadi R. Critical care management of

potential organ donors: Our current standard. Clin Transplant 2009; 23 (Suppl. 21): 2-9.
[http://dx.doi.org/10.1111/j.1399-0012.2009.01102.x]

[45]   Matesanz R, Dominguez-Gil B. Strategies to optimize deceased organ donation. Transplant Rev (Orlando) 2007; 21: 177-88.
[http://dx.doi.org/10.1016/j.trre.2007.07.005]

[46]   Matesanz R, Miranda B, Felipe C. Organ procurement in Spain: impact of transplant coordination. Clin Transplant 1994; 8: 281-6.

[47]   Matesanz R, Miranda B, Felipe C. Organ procurement and renal transplants in Spain: the impact of transplant coordination. Nephrol Dial Transplant 1994; 9: 475-8.
[http://dx.doi.org/10.1093/ndt/9.5.475]

[48]   Matesanz R. Factors influencing the adaptation of the Spanish Model of organ donation. Transpl Int 2003; 16: 736-41.
[http://dx.doi.org/10.1111/j.1432-2277.2003.tb00233.x]

[49]   Manyalich M, Cabrer C, Vilardell J, Miranda B. Functions, responsibilities, dedication, payment, organization, and profile of the hospital transplant coordination in Spain in 2002. Transplant Proc 2003; 35: 1633-5.
[http://dx.doi.org/10.1016/S0041-1345(03)00694-8]

[50]   Páez G, Valero R, Paredes D, *et al.* Evaluation of transplant procurement management courses: An educational project as a tool for the optimization of transplant coordination. Transplant Proc 2003; 35: 1638-9.
[http://dx.doi.org/10.1016/S0041-1345(03)00695-X]

[51]   Rodriguez-Arias D, Wright L, Paredes D. Success factors and ethical challenges of the Spanish Model of organ donation. Lancet 2010; 376: 1109-12.
[http://dx.doi.org/10.1016/S0140-6736(10)61342-6]

[52]   Council of Europe. International Figures on donation and transplantation - 2015. Newsl Transpl 2016; p. 21.

[53]   Marks WH, Wagner D, Pearson TC, *et al.* Organ donation and utilization, 1995-2004: Entering the collaborative era. Am J Transplant 2006; 6: 1101-10.
[http://dx.doi.org/10.1111/j.1600-6143.2006.01269.x]

[54]   Duda L. Virtual Mentor, September 2005 Virtual Mentor Health Law National Organ Allocation Policy: The Final Rule. Ethics J Am Med Assoc 2005; 7(9)

[55]   Health Resources and Services Administration (HRSA), Department of Health and Human Services (HHS). Organ procurement and transplantation network. Final rule. Fed Regist 2013; 78(128): 40033-42.

[56]   De Carlis L, Sguinzi R, Grande A, Aseni P. Multiple organ retrieval: general principles, organ preservation, and new strategies.Multiorgan Procurement for Transplantation. Cham: Springer International Publishing 2016; pp. 79-90.
[http://dx.doi.org/10.1007/978-3-319-28416-3_8]

CHAPTER 6

Current State of Organ Preservation

Eliza Beal, Bryan Whitson* and **Sylvester Black**

The Ohio State University, Columbus, OH, USA

Abstract: The objective of this chapter is to review the principles of organ preservation and current preservation solutions employed in multi-organ transplantation with specific reference to unique organ specific preservation.

Keywords: Multi-Organ Transplantation, Organ Preservation.

INTRODUCTION

Organ preservation is a critical component of the transplantation process, potentially contributing to improved graft and patient outcomes. Preservation solutions are designed to mitigate cellular injury during procurement and transport. Each organ type has a different cellular composition and metabolic needs and likely requires a different preservation solution. Delayed graft function and potential graft failure are possible consequences of inadequate preservation and confer significant risk of morbidity and mortality for the patient [1].

Initial efforts at organ preservation were aimed at reducing the accumulation of harmful toxins during ischemia and incorporated hypothermia, which showed to maintain a baseline level of metabolism, but reduce tissue oxygenation and minimize tissue damage [2, 3]. Hypothermia has the potential to cause significant cell damage, inducing mitochondrial dysfunction, disruption of ion channel function and calcium homeostasis, reduction of adenosine triphosphate (ATP), and accumulation of xanthine oxidase and reactive oxygen species [4]. This led to the development of preservation solutions, which were incorporated into mainstream graft preservation techniques.

Current preservation solutions contain differing combinations of impermeants, buffers, antioxidants and energy substrates aimed at maximizing graft function and survival [1, 5]. Collins solution, introduced in the late 1960's, increased cold storage time of the kidney from 12 to 30 hours and contained a combination of

* **Corresponding author Bryan Whitson:** The Ohio State University, Columbus, OH, USA; Tel: 614-293-8000; Email: bryan.whitson@osumc.edu

Robert S.D. Higgins & Juan A. Sanchez (Eds.)

mannitol, phenoxybenzamine, procaine, glucose, heparin, KH_2PO_4, K_2HPO_4, KCL, $NaHCO_3$, and $MgSO_4$ [6]. Phenoxybenzamine, procaine, heparin and magnesium phosphate were removed to form Euro-Collins, a modified Collins solution, after it was found that heparin and phenoxybenazamine were non-essential, procaine was nephrotoxic and magnesium phosphate was prone to crystallization [7, 8]. Belzer solution, another early preservation solution, contained thawed AB^+ or AB^- plasma, distilled water, KCL and mannitol, penicillin, decadron, $MgSO_4$ and insulin [9]. An early study demonstrated improved graft and patient survival with Collins solution in comparison to Belzer solution and Euro-Collins solution which is widely used [10].

In the late 1980s, additional preservation solutions were introduced including histidine-tryptophan-ketoglutarate (HTK), University of Wisconsin (UW) solution and Celsior [11 - 13]. The University of Wisconsin solution was shown to be effective for liver graft preservation with ischemic times greater than 8 hours and for combined renal-pancreas and isolated pancreas grafts with ischemic times up to 19 hours [12, 14]. It was later demonstrated that high molecular weight components of UW including hydroethyl starch, made the solution viscous, and it was implicated in graft dysfunction [15]. Less viscous solutions including Celsior and HTK then gained popularity. HTK was introduced in 1989 in liver graft preservation [13]. Celsior was first used in cardiac grafts and was later adopted in the liver, renal and pancreas preservation [16 - 20].

Efforts have also been made to specifically target cardiac and pulmonary organ preservation. Plegisol and Papworth were introduced as preservation solutions for cardiac grafts [21, 22]. Perfadex was designed specifically for pulmonary preservation and is FDA approved only for that indication [5].

Clear consensus on which preservation solution is optimal for each indication has not been achieved – it has been reported that on surveying United Network for Organ Sharing cardiac transplant centers, the use of 167 different solutions was observed [23].

Preservation Solutions

Classification of Preservation Solutions

Current preservation solutions contain different combinations of impermeants, buffers, antioxidants and energy substrates aimed at maximizing graft function and survival [1, 5]. Several preservation solutions for abdominal and thoracic transplant are compared in Table **6.1**.

Intracellular Vs. Extracellular Solutions

Euro-Collins and University of Wisconsin solutions were designed to replicate the intracellular environment and have low sodium and high potassium concentrations [23, 24] in an effort to mitigate the consequences of hypothermia induced sodium-potassium transmembrane pump dysfunction. However, these solutions carry an increased risk of vasospasm and endothelial dysfunction [25 - 28]. Newer strategies include low sodium, low potassium solutions such as HTK or high sodium, low potassium solutions such as Celsior, Perfadex, Papworth and Plegisol, although it has been concluded that both strategies are equally effective [26, 29].

Impermeants

Impermeants and colloids are used to combat cellular edema, which lead to reduced tolerance to anoxia [30]. Impermeants in use include glucose, mannitol, lactobionate, raffinose and hydroxyethyl starch [12, 30, 31]. Impermeant contents of current preservation solutions are demonstrated in Table **6.1**.

Table 6.1. Comparison of Select Perfusate Solutions*,**.

	EC	UW	HTK	Celsior	Per	Papworth	Plegisol
Study	Aziz [34]	Roskott [33]	Roskott [33], 't Hart [89]	Roskott [33], t' Hart [89]	Aziz [34]	Marasco [81], Divisi [22]	Chambers [21]
IC/EX	IC	IC	EX	EX	EX	EX	EX
Na$^+$	10	25	15	100	138	115	120
K$^+$	115	120	10	15	6	3	16
Impermeant/Colloid	Glucose	LactoB, raffinose, HES	Mannitol	LactoB, Mannitol	Dextran	Mannitol, albumin	N/A
Buffer	Phos, Bicarb	Phos	Histidine	Histidine	Phos	N/A	Bicarb
Antioxidant	N/A	AlloP, GSH	Trp, Mannitol	GSH, Mannitol	N/A	Mannitol	N/A
Osmolarity (mOsm/L)	375	330	310	320	292	440	320
Ca2$^+$	N/A	N/A	0.02	0.25	N/A	Undetermined	1.2
Mg2$^+$	N/A	5	4	13	0.8	N/A	16
Cl$^-$	15	20	32	N/A	142	Undetermined	160
Glucose	180	N/A	N/A	N/A	5	N/A	N/A

(Table 6.1) cont.....

	EC	UW	HTK	Celsior	Per	Papworth	Plegisol
Others	N/A	Adenosine, Insulin, Dexamethasone	Glutamate, Alpha-ketoglutarate	Glutamate	SO42⁻ 0.8, Dextran 40 g/L	Donor blood, Heparin	N/A

*All units expressed in mmol/L unless otherwise indicated. Abbreviations: IC, intracellular; EX, extracellular; EC, Euro Collins; UW, University of Wisconsin; HTK, histidine-tryptophan-ketoglutarate; CEL, Celsior; PER, Perfadex; Und, undetermined; LactoB, lactobionate; HES, hydroxyethyl starch; Phos, phosphate; Bicarb, bicarbonate; GSH, glutathione; AlloP, allopurinol; Trp, tryptophan.

**Adapted From: Latchana N, Peck JR, Whitson B, Black SM. Preservation solutions for cardiac and pulmonary donor grafts: a review of the current literature. J Thorac Dis. 2014 Aug;6(8):1143-9. doi: 10.3978/j.issn.2072-1439.2014.05.14 and Latchana N, Peck JR, Whitson BA, Henry ML, Elkhammas EA, Black SM. Preservation solutions used during abdominal transplantation: Current status and outcomes. World J Transplant 2015; 5(4): 154-164 Available from: URL: http://www.wjgnet.com/2220-3230/full/v5/i4/154.htm DOI: http://dx.doi.org/10.5500/wjt.v5.i4.154.*

Antioxidants

Oxygen free radicals generated during reperfusion injury lead to lipid peroxidation of cell membranes, production of malondialdehyde and cell death and their inclusion in preservation solutions can alleviate damage [32]. Allopurinol, a xanthine oxidase inhibitor, and glutathione, a reducing agent, were included in UW solution and further attempts at including antioxidants have been made [26, 33].

Buffers

Anaerobic metabolism and ATP hydrolysis during graft ischemia lead to metabolic acidosis and cellular dysfunction [34, 35]. Inclusion of buffers in preservation solutions can maintain physiologic pH [35, 36].

Energy Precursors

Energy precursors included in preservation solutions lead to increased levels of adenosine triphosphate (ATP) during ischemia reperfusion, which contributes to improved mitochondrial function [31].

Abdominal Transplant

Liver Preservation

Studies comparing preservation solutions used for liver preservation, including UW, HTK and Celsior, have been performed. No difference in patient, or graft, survival in comparing UW to HTK or Celsior to UW or HTK has been demonstrated [37 - 43]. Similarity in graft and patient survival between UW and HTK has also been demonstrated in extended-criteria donor and living donor transplantation and a meta-analysis performed by Feng *et al* including 1200 patients demonstrated no difference between the two solutions [41, 44 - 46]. Although graft and patient outcomes are similar with the use of UW and HTK, it has been shown that the use of HTK leads to substantial cost savings [39, 44, 45, 47]. Similarly no differences in patient or graft survival have been found in comparing Celsior to UW or HTK in prospective studies or randomized controlled trials [48 - 52].

Some studies have demonstrated superiority of HTK to UW in terms of biliary complications [15, 39, 43]. A retrospective study of 256 liver transplants demonstrated that HTK was superior to UW in protecting against the formation of biliary anastomotic strictures (OR = 0.40, p=0.0005) [15]. HTK has been demonstrated to result in reduced incidence of biliary sludge [39]. Other studies have failed to demonstrate a difference in biliary complications between UW and HTK [38, 40, 53].

In summary, although the evidence is certainly not conclusive, the potential cost-savings and reduced biliary complications associated with HTK make it an enticing choice for use in liver transplantation.

Renal Preservation

The use of UW and HTK in renal preservation has also been explored. Similar rates of graft and patient survival between UW and HTK have been demonstrated [54 - 56]. In initial studies, UW led to increased incidence of delayed graft function in living donor transplants (UW 8.2% vs, HTK 3.2%, p=0.001) and HTK led to increased incidence of delayed graft function in deceased donor transplants (UW 17.4% vs. HTK 26.2%, p=0.005) but further multi-center randomized controlled trials have demonstrated similar graft and patient survival, and similar rates of delayed graft function in comparing UW and HTK [54 - 56]. Cost-savings have also been noted with the use of HTK in renal preservation [57, 58]. The use of Celsior in renal preservation has also been investigated with no differences in graft or patient survival, or in graft dysfunction [18, 51, 59]. In summary, UW, HTK and Celsior are likely comparable in terms of patient and graft survival and delayed graft function. The use of HTK may be preferable given the potential cost savings.

Pancreas Preservation

UW has been compared to both HTK and Celsior in pancreas preservation and graft and patient survival are similar [20, 60 - 66], however it has been suggested in small studies that HTK may lead to increased rates of graft thrombosis and pancreatitis [64, 65, 67], but this finding was not confirmed in larger studies [68].

HTK may also be more cost effective for pancreas graft preservation [61, 65, 69]. In comparing UW and Celsior, it has been demonstrated that there is no difference in graft or patient survival [20, 66]. UW and Celsior are adequate preservation solutions for use in pancreas transplantation. The possible association of HTK with pancreatitis and graft thrombosis suggests that further studies should be performed.

Intestinal Preservation

There are few studies to guide choice of preservation solution in intestinal transplantation. Graft ischemia in intestinal transplantation is limited to 6 to 10 hours and UW has been shown to be less effective than in other abdominal organs [33]. Both intravascular and intraluminal flushes have been proposed to improve mucosal integrity and reduce bacterial translocation [33, 70].

Cardiac and Pulmonary Transplant

Heart Transplantation

Cold ischemia times for cardiac transplantation as long as 13 hours have been reported, but are usually limited to less than 6 hours [71, 72]. Celsior was reported to be an effective preservation solution for cardiac transplantation and several studies have supported its use [73 - 76]. In comparing UW to HTK it was noted that there was a survival benefit with the use of UW and George *et al.,* performed a study of 4,910 patients (UW 3,107 and Celsior 1,803) that revealed higher 1-year survival in the UW group (UW 89.6% vs. Celsior 87.0%, p<0.01) [77, 78]. These studies suggest that UW is the optimal preservation solution for cardiac transplantation among those currently available. The use of heart perfusion systems is currently under investigation (Fig. **6.1**).

Lung Transplantation

The lung is very sensitive to ischemia reperfusion injury and can only tolerate ischemic periods up to 6 hours [79]. EC, Papworth and Perfadex are common preservation solutions for lung transplantation. In 157 lung transplants using EC, Papworth or Perfadex there was no difference in 30-day mortality between groups [80], but a follow-up study at the same institution demonstrated a correlation with long-term risk of death associated with the use of Papworth versus EC or Perfadex in 310 patients [81]. Both of these studies demonstrated lower incidence of primary graft dysfunction with Perfadex [80, 81]. EC and Perfadex and EC and UW have been found to be comparable in some studies, while others demonstrate increased duration of mechanical ventilation and improved PaO2/FiO2 ratio with the use of Perfadex [34, 82 - 88]. In summary, there appears to be sufficient evidence to warn against the use of Papworth and UW. In comparing EC and Perfadex, there does not appear to be a mortality advantage, but the improved PaO_2/FiO_2 ratio and lower duration of mechanical ventilation support the of Perfadex.

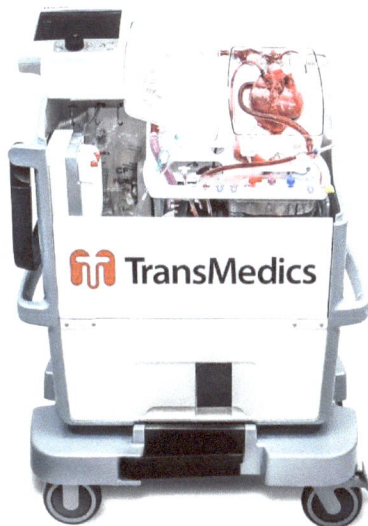

Fig. (6.1). Transmedics OCS Heart. Used with permission. Medical Illustrations© 2018 Tim Phelps, MS, FAMI, Johns Hopkins University.

CONCLUSION

In liver transplantation some benefit of histidine-tryptophan-ketoglutarate (HTK) over the University of Wisconsin solution has been demonstrated in terms of biliary complications and cost. The use of Euro-Collins in renal preservation may lead to increased graft dysfunction. Additionally, the use of HTK can lead to substantial cost savings. In pancreas transplantation the use of University of Wisconsin solution and Celsior are common. HTK has been shown to be associated with pancreatitis and graft thrombosis. However, no difference in graft or patient survival has been demonstrated between different preservation solutions in liver, renal or pancreas transplantation. Limited evidence on preservation for intestinal transplantation has been generated. The use of intraluminal University of Wisconsin solution with an intra-vascular washout has been recommended [1]. UW solution is the preservation solution of choice for cardiac transplants. Despite this success, outcomes with UW are more disappointing for lung transplantation and perfadex may be preferable.

CONSENT FOR PUBLICATION

Not applicable.

CONFLICT OF INTEREST

The author declares no conflict of interest, financial or otherwise.

ACKNOWLEDGEMENTS

Declared none.

REFERENCES

[1]   Latchana N, Peck JR, Whitson BA, Henry ML, Elkhammas EA, Black SM. Preservation solutions used during abdominal transplantation: Current status and outcomes. World J Transplant 2015; 5(4): 154-64.
[http://dx.doi.org/10.5500/wjt.v5.i4.154]

[2]   Hartley LC, Collins GM, Clunie GJ. Kidney preservation for transportation. Function of 29 human-cadaver kidneys preserved with an intracellular perfusate. N Engl J Med 1971; 285(19): 1049-52.
[http://dx.doi.org/10.1056/NEJM197111042851903]

[3]   Lillehei RC, Manax WG, Bloch JH, Eyal Z, Hidalgo F, Longerbeam JK. *In vitro* preservation of whole organs by hypothermia and hyperbaric oxygenation. Cryobiology 1964; 1(2): 181-93.

[4]   Guibert EE, Petrenko AY, Balaban CL, Somov AY, Rodriguez JV, Fuller BJ. Organ preservation: current concepts and new strategies for the next decade. Transfus Med Hemother 2011; 38(2): 125-42.
[http://dx.doi.org/10.1159/000327033]

[5]   Latchana N, Peck JR, Whitson B, Black SM. Preservation solutions for cardiac and pulmonary donor grafts: a review of the current literature. J Thorac Dis 2014; 6(8): 1143-9.

[6]   Collins GM, Bravo-Shugarman M, Terasaki PI. Kidney preservation for transportation. Initial perfusion and 30 hours' ice storage. Lancet 1969; 2(7632): 1219-22.
[http://dx.doi.org/10.1016/S0140-6736(69)90753-3]

[7]   Collins GM, Halasz NA. Letter: Composition of intracellular flush solutions for hypothermic kidney storage. Lancet 1975; 1(7900): 220.

[8]   Dreikorn K, Horsch R, Röhl L. 48- to 96-hour preservation of canine kidneys by initial perfusion and hypothermic storage using the Euro-Collins solution. Eur Urol 1980; 6(4): 221-4.
[http://dx.doi.org/10.1159/000473336]

[9]   Belzer FO, Kountz SL. Preservation and transplantation of human cadaver kidneys: a two-year experience. Ann Surg 1970; 172(3): 394-404.
[http://dx.doi.org/10.1097/00000658-197009000-00009]

[10]   Clark EA, Opelz G, Mickey MR, Terasaki PI. Evaluation of Belzer and Collins kidney-preservation methods. Lancet 1973; 1(7799): 361-4.
[http://dx.doi.org/10.1016/S0140-6736(73)90142-6]

[11]   Gubernatis G, Pichlmayr R, Lamesch P, *et al.* HTK-solution (Bretschneider) for human liver transplantation. First clinical experiences. Langenbecks Arch Chir 1990; 375(2): 66-70.
[http://dx.doi.org/10.1007/BF00713388]

[12]   Kalayoglu M, Sollinger HW, Stratta RJ, *et al.* Extended preservation of the liver for clinical transplantation. Lancet 1988; 1(8586): 617-9.

[13]   Feng XN, Xu X, Zheng SS. Current status and perspective of liver preservation solutions. Hepatobiliary Pancreat Dis Int 2006; 5(4): 490-4.

[14]   D'Alessandro AM, Stratta RJ, Sollinger HW, Kalayoglu M, Pirsch JD, Belzer FO. Use of UW solution in pancreas transplantation. Diabetes 1989; 38 (Suppl. 1): 7-9.
[http://dx.doi.org/10.2337/diab.38.1.S7]

[15]   Welling TH, Heidt DG, Englesbe MJ, *et al.* Biliary complications following liver transplantation in the model for end-stage liver disease era: effect of donor, recipient, and technical factors. Liver Transpl 2008; 14(1): 73-80.
[http://dx.doi.org/10.1002/lt.21354]

[16]   Biernat M, Garlicki M, Dziatkowiak A. Correlation between heart rate variability and hypothermic storage in human cardiac transplant recipients. Ann Transplant 1998; 3(4): 37-40.

[17]   Maggi U, Caccamo L, Gatti S, *et al.* Celsior solution and clinical liver transplantation. Transplant Proc 2000; 32(1): 36-7.
[http://dx.doi.org/10.1016/S0041-1345(99)00866-0]

[18]   Faenza A, Catena F, Nardo B, *et al.* Kidney preservation with university of Wisconsin and Celsior solution: a prospective multicenter randomized study. Transplantation 2001; 72(7): 1274-7.
[http://dx.doi.org/10.1097/00007890-200110150-00016]

[19]   Karam G, Compagnon P, Hourmant M, *et al.* A single solution for multiple organ procurement and preservation. Transpl Int 2005; 18(6): 657-63.
[http://dx.doi.org/10.1111/j.1432-2277.2005.00083.x]

[20]   Boggi U, Coletti L, Vistoli F, *et al.* Pancreas preservation with University of Wisconsin and Celsior solutions. Transplant Proc 2004; 36(3): 563-5.
[http://dx.doi.org/10.1016/j.transproceed.2004.03.078]

[21]   Chambers DJ, Sakai A, Braimbridge MV, *et al.* Clinical validation of St. Thomas' Hospital cardioplegic solution No. 2 (Plegisol). Eur J Cardiothorac Surg 1989; 3(4): 346-52.
[http://dx.doi.org/10.1016/1010-7940(89)90033-X]

[22]   Divisi D, Montagna P, Jegaden O, *et al.* A comparative study of Euro-Collins, low potassium University of Wisconsin and cold modified blood solutions in lung preservation in acute autotransplantations in the pig. Eur J Cardiothorac Surg 2001; 19(3): 333-8.
[http://dx.doi.org/10.1016/S1010-7940(00)00656-4]

[23]   Demmy TL, Biddle JS, Bennett LE, Walls JT, Schmaltz RA, Curtis JJ. Organ preservation solutions in heart transplantation-patterns of usage and related survival. Transplantation 1997; 63(2): 262-9.
[http://dx.doi.org/10.1097/00007890-199701270-00015]

[24]   Abouna GM, Hurwitz R, Serrou B. Organ preservation by Collins' solution. Lancet 1971; 1(7708): 1076.
[http://dx.doi.org/10.1016/S0140-6736(71)91646-1]

[25]   Fukuse T, Albes JM, Brandes H, Takahashi Y, Demertzis S, Schäfers HJ. Comparison of low potassium Euro-Collins solution and standard Euro-Collins solution in an extracorporeal rat heart-lung model. Eur J Cardiothorac Surg 1996; 10(8): 621-7.
[http://dx.doi.org/10.1016/S1010-7940(96)80376-9]

[26]   Collins GM, Wicomb WN. New organ preservation solutions. Kidney Int Suppl 1992; 38: S197-202.

[27]   Warnecke G, Strüber M, Hohlfeld JM, Niedermeyer J, Sommer SP, Haverich A. Pulmonary preservation with Bretscheider's HTK and Celsior solution in minipigs. Eur J Cardiothorac Surg 2002; 21(6): 1073-9.
[http://dx.doi.org/10.1016/S1010-7940(02)00106-9]

[28]   Featherstone RL, Kelly FJ, Shattock MJ, Hearse DJ, Chambers DJ. Hypothermic preservation of isolated rat lungs in modified bicarbonate buffer, EuroCollins solution or St Thomas' Hospital cardioplegic solution. Eur J Cardiothorac Surg 1998; 14(5): 508-15.
[http://dx.doi.org/10.1016/S1010-7940(98)00188-2]

[29]   't Hart NA, der van Plaats A, Leuvenink HG, *et al.* Determination of an adequate perfusion pressure for continuous dual vessel hypothermic machine perfusion of the rat liver. Transpl Int 2007; 20(4): 343-52.
[http://dx.doi.org/10.1111/j.1432-2277.2006.00433.x]

[30]   Jamart J, Lambotte L. Efficiency and limitation of Euro-Collins solution in kidney preservation. J Surg Res 1983; 34(3): 195-204.
[http://dx.doi.org/10.1016/0022-4804(83)90060-4]

[31]   Janssen H, Janssen PH, Broelsch CE. Celsior solution compared with University of Wisconsin solution (UW) and histidine-tryptophan-ketoglutarate solution (HTK) in the protection of human hepatocytes against ischemia-reperfusion injury. Transpl Int 2003; 16(7): 515-22.

[32]   Marzi I, Zhi ZN, Zimmermann FA, Lemasters JJ, Thurman RG. Xanthine and hypoxanthine accumulation during storage may contribute to reperfusion injury following liver transplantation in the rat. Transplant Proc 1989; 21(1 Pt 2): 1319-20.

[33]   Roskott AM, Nieuwenhuijs VB, Dijkstra G, Koudstaal LG, Leuvenink HG, Ploeg RJ. Small bowel preservation for intestinal transplantation: a review. Transpl Int 2011; 24(2): 107-31.
[http://dx.doi.org/10.1111/j.1432-2277.2010.01187.x]

[34]   Aziz TM, Pillay TM, Corris PA, *et al.* Perfadex for clinical lung procurement: is it an advance? Ann Thorac Surg 2003; 75(3): 990-5.
[http://dx.doi.org/10.1016/S0003-4975(02)04491-0]

[35]   Sumimoto R, Kamada N, Jamieson NV, Fukuda Y, Dohi K. A comparison of a new solution combining histidine and lactobionate with UW solution and eurocollins for rat liver preservation. Transplantation 1991; 51(3): 589-93.
[http://dx.doi.org/10.1097/00007890-199103000-00010]

[36]   Schilling M, Redaelli C, Friess H, Laeuffer J, Büchler M. Temperature dependence of proton buffering capacity of HTK, Euro-Collins, and UW solution. Transplant Proc 1996; 28(1): 343-4.

[37]   Pokorny H, Rasoul-Rockenschaub S, Langer F, *et al.* Histidine-tryptophan-ketoglutarate solution for organ preservation in human liver transplantation-a prospective multi-centre observation study. Transpl Int 2004; 17(5): 256-60.
[http://dx.doi.org/10.1111/j.1432-2277.2004.tb00439.x]

[38]   Erhard J, Lange R, Scherer R, *et al.* Comparison of histidine-tryptophan-ketoglutarate (HTK) solution versus University of Wisconsin (UW) solution for organ preservation in human liver transplantation. A prospective, randomized study. Transpl Int 1994; 7(3): 177-81.

[39]   Mangus RS, Tector AJ, Agarwal A, Vianna R, Murdock P, Fridell JA. Comparison of histidine-tryptophan-ketoglutarate solution (HTK) and University of Wisconsin solution (UW) in adult liver transplantation. Liver Transpl 2006; 12(2): 226-30.
[http://dx.doi.org/10.1002/lt.20552]

[40]   Rayya F, Harms J, Martin AP, Bartels M, Hauss J, Fangmann J. Comparison of histidine-tryptopha--ketoglutarate solution and University of Wisconsin solution in adult liver transplantation. Transplant Proc 2008; 40(4): 891-4.
[http://dx.doi.org/10.1016/j.transproceed.2008.03.044]

[41]   Mangus RS, Fridell JA, Vianna RM, *et al.* Comparison of histidine-tryptophan-ketoglutarate solution and University of Wisconsin solution in extended criteria liver donors. Liver Transpl 2008; 14(3): 365-73.
[http://dx.doi.org/10.1002/lt.21372]

[42]   Avolio AW, Agnes S, Nure E, *et al.* Comparative evaluation of two perfusion solutions for liver preservation and transplantation. Transplant Proc 2006; 38(4): 1066-7.
[http://dx.doi.org/10.1016/j.transproceed.2006.03.009]

[43]   Canelo R, Hakim NS, Ringe B. Experience with hystidine tryptophan ketoglutarate versus University Wisconsin preservation solutions in transplantation. Int Surg 2003; 88(3): 145-51.

[44]   Chan SC, Liu CL, Lo CM, Fan ST. Applicability of histidine-tryptophan-ketoglutarate solution in right lobe adult-to-adult live donor liver transplantation. Liver Transpl 2004; 10(11): 1415-21.
[http://dx.doi.org/10.1002/lt.20243]

[45]   Testa G, Malagó M, Nadalin S, *et al.* Histidine-tryptophan-ketoglutarate versus University of Wisconsin solution in living donor liver transplantation: results of a prospective study. Liver Transpl 2003; 9(8): 822-6.
[http://dx.doi.org/10.1053/jlts.2003.50168]

[46]   Feng L, Zhao N, Yao X, *et al.* Histidine-tryptophan-ketoglutarate solution vs. University of Wisconsin solution for liver transplantation: a systematic review. Liver Transpl 2007; 13(8): 1125-36.
[http://dx.doi.org/10.1002/lt.21208]

[47]   Ringe B, Braun F, Moritz M, Zeldin G, Soriano H, Meyers W. Safety and efficacy of living donor liver preservation with HTK solution. Transplant Proc 2005; 37(1): 316-9.

[48]   Lopez-Andujar R, Deusa S, Montalvá E, *et al.* Comparative prospective study of two liver graft preservation solutions: University of Wisconsin and Celsior. Liver Transpl 2009; 15(12): 1709-17.
[http://dx.doi.org/10.1002/lt.21945]

[49]   García-Gil FA, Arenas J, Güemes A, *et al.* Preservation of the liver graft with Celsior solution. Transplant Proc 2006; 38(8): 2385-8.
[http://dx.doi.org/10.1016/j.transproceed.2006.08.032]

[50]   Cavallari A, Cillo U, Nardo B, *et al.* A multicenter pilot prospective study comparing Celsior and University of Wisconsin preserving solutions for use in liver transplantation. Liver Transpl 2003; 9(8): 814-21.
[http://dx.doi.org/10.1053/jlts.2003.50161]

[51]   Pedotti P, Cardillo M, Rigotti P, *et al.* A comparative prospective study of two available solutions for kidney and liver preservation. Transplantation 2004; 77(10): 1540-5.
[http://dx.doi.org/10.1097/01.TP.0000132278.00441.CF]

[52]   Nardo B, Bertelli R, Montalti R, *et al.* Preliminary results of a clinical randomized study comparing Celsior and HTK solutions in liver preservation for transplantation. Transplant Proc 2005; 37(1): 320-2.
[http://dx.doi.org/10.1016/j.transproceed.2004.11.028]

[53]   Moench C, Otto G. Ischemic type biliary lesions in histidine-tryptophan-ketoglutarate (HTK) preserved liver grafts. Int J Artif Organs 2006; 29(3): 329-34.
[http://dx.doi.org/10.1177/039139880602900311]

[54]   Lynch RJ, Kubus J, Chenault RH, Pelletier SJ, Campbell DA, Englesbe MJ. Comparison of histidine-tryptophan-ketoglutarate and University of Wisconsin preservation in renal transplantation. Am J Transplant 2008; 8(3): 567-73.
[http://dx.doi.org/10.1111/j.1600-6143.2007.02065.x]

[55]   de Boer J, De Meester J, Smits JM, *et al.* Eurotransplant randomized multicenter kidney graft preservation study comparing HTK with UW and Euro-Collins. Transpl Int 1999; 12(6): 447-53.
[http://dx.doi.org/10.1007/s001470050256]

[56]   Klaus F, Castro DB, Bittar CM, *et al.* Kidney transplantation with Belzer or Custodiol solution: a randomized prospective study. Transplant Proc 2007; 39(2): 353-4.
[http://dx.doi.org/10.1016/j.transproceed.2007.01.009]

[57]   Englesbe MJ, Heidt D, Sung R, Pietroski R. Does using HTK solution for cold perfusion of cadaveric kidneys save money? Transplantation 2006; 81(12): 1750.
[http://dx.doi.org/10.1097/01.tp.0000226079.94635.3f]

[58]   Moray G, Sevmis S, Karakayali FY, Gorur SK, Haberal M. Comparison of histidine-tryptopha-ketoglutarate and University of Wisconsin in living-donor liver transplantation. Transplant Proc 2006; 38(10): 3572-5.
[http://dx.doi.org/10.1016/j.transproceed.2006.10.174]

[59]   Montalti R, Nardo B, Capocasale E, *et al.* Kidney transplantation from elderly donors: a prospective randomized study comparing celsior and UW solutions. Transplant Proc 2005; 37(6): 2454-5.

[http://dx.doi.org/10.1016/j.transproceed.2005.06.030]

[60]   Potdar S, Malek S, Eghtesad B, *et al.* Initial experience using histidine-tryptophan-ketoglutarate solution in clinical pancreas transplantation. Clin Transplant 2004; 18(6): 661-5.
[http://dx.doi.org/10.1111/j.1399-0012.2004.00262.x]

[61]   Englesbe MJ, Moyer A, Kim DY, *et al.* Early pancreas transplant outcomes with histidine-tryptopha--ketoglutarate preservation: a multicenter study. Transplantation 2006; 82(1): 136-9.
[http://dx.doi.org/10.1097/01.tp.0000225764.21343.e3]

[62]   Schneeberger S, Biebl M, Steurer W, *et al.* A prospective randomized multicenter trial comparing histidine-tryptophane-ketoglutarate versus University of Wisconsin perfusion solution in clinical pancreas transplantation. Transpl Int 2009; 22(2): 217-24.
[http://dx.doi.org/10.1111/j.1432-2277.2008.00773.x]

[63]   Becker T, Ringe B, Nyibata M, *et al.* Pancreas transplantation with histidine-tryptophan-ketoglutarate (HTK) solution and University of Wisconsin (UW) solution: is there a difference? JOP 2007; 8(3): 304-11.

[64]   Agarwal A, Powelson JA, Goggins WC, Milgrom ML, Fridell JA. Organ preservation with histidine-tryptophan ketogluatarate solution in clinical pancreas transplantation: an update of the indiana university experience. Transplant Proc 2008; 40(2): 498-501.
[http://dx.doi.org/10.1016/j.transproceed.2008.01.011]

[65]   Alonso D, Dunn TB, Rigley T, *et al.* Increased pancreatitis in allografts flushed with histidine-tryptophan-ketoglutarate solution: a cautionary tale. Am J Transplant 2008; 8(9): 1942-5.
[http://dx.doi.org/10.1111/j.1600-6143.2008.02312.x]

[66]   Manrique A, Jiménez C, Herrero ML, *et al.* Pancreas preservation with the University of Wisconsin versus Celsior solutions. Transplant Proc 2006; 38(8): 2582-4.
[http://dx.doi.org/10.1016/j.transproceed.2006.08.058]

[67]   Agarwal A, Murdock P, Pescovitz MD, Goggins WC, Milgrom ML, Fridell JA. Follow-up experience using histidine-tryptophan ketoglutarate solution in clinical pancreas transplantation. Transplant Proc 2005; 37(8): 3523-6.
[http://dx.doi.org/10.1016/j.transproceed.2005.09.069]

[68]   Fridell JA, Mangus RS, Powelson JA. Histidine-tryptophan-ketoglutarate for pancreas allograft preservation: the Indiana University experience. Am J Transplant 2010; 10(5): 1284-9.
[http://dx.doi.org/10.1111/j.1600-6143.2010.03095.x]

[69]   Bellamy CA, Nicely B, Mattice BJ, Teaster R. Comparative analysis of clinical efficacy and cost between University of Wisconsin solution and histidine-tryptophan-ketoglutarate. Prog Transplant 2008; 18(3): 166-71.
[http://dx.doi.org/10.1177/152692480801800304]

[70]   Oltean M, Churchill TA. Organ-specific solutions and strategies for the intestinal preservation. Int Rev Immunol 2014; 33(3): 234-44.
[http://dx.doi.org/10.3109/08830185.2013.853764]

[71]   Wei J, Chang CY, Chuang YC, *et al.* Successful heart transplantation after 13 hours of donor heart ischemia with the use of HTK solution: a case report. Transplant Proc 2005; 37(5): 2253-4.
[http://dx.doi.org/10.1016/j.transproceed.2005.03.055]

[72]   Southard JH, Belzer FO. Organ preservation. Annu Rev Med 1995; 46: 235-47.
[http://dx.doi.org/10.1146/annurev.med.46.1.235]

[73]   Remadi JP, Baron O, Roussel JC, *et al.* Myocardial preservation using Celsior solution in cardiac transplantation: early results and 5-year follow-up of a multicenter prospective study of 70 cardiac transplantations. Ann Thorac Surg 2002; 73(5): 1495-9.
[http://dx.doi.org/10.1016/S0003-4975(02)03424-0]

[74]   De Santo LS, Amarelli C, Romano G, *et al.* High-risk heart grafts: effective preservation with Celsior

solution. Heart Vessels 2006; 21(2): 89-94.
[http://dx.doi.org/10.1007/s00380-005-0867-z]

[75]   Wieselthaler GM, Chevtchik O, Konetschny R, *et al.* Improved graft function using a new myocardial preservation solution: Celsior. Preliminary data from a randomized prospective study. Transplant Proc 1999; 31(5): 2067-8.
[http://dx.doi.org/10.1016/S0041-1345(99)00264-X]

[76]   Vega JD, Ochsner JL, Jeevanandam V, *et al.* A multicenter, randomized, controlled trial of Celsior for flush and hypothermic storage of cardiac allografts. Ann Thorac Surg 2001; 71(5): 1442-7.
[http://dx.doi.org/10.1016/S0003-4975(01)02458-4]

[77]   Kofler S, Bigdeli AK, Kaczmarek I, *et al.* Long-term outcomes after 1000 heart transplantations in six different eras of innovation in a single center. Transpl Int 2009; 22(12): 1140-50.
[http://dx.doi.org/10.1111/j.1432-2277.2009.00931.x]

[78]   George TJ, Arnaoutakis GJ, Baumgartner WA, Shah AS, Conte JV. Organ storage with University of Wisconsin solution is associated with improved outcomes after orthotopic heart transplantation. J Heart Lung Transplant 2011; 30(9): 1033-43.
[http://dx.doi.org/10.1016/j.healun.2011.05.005]

[79]   Arcasoy SM, Kotloff RM. Lung transplantation. N Engl J Med 1999; 340(14): 1081-91.
[http://dx.doi.org/10.1056/NEJM199904083401406]

[80]   Oto T, Griffiths AP, Rosenfeldt F, Levvey BJ, Williams TJ, Snell GI. Early outcomes comparing Perfadex, Euro-Collins, and Papworth solutions in lung transplantation. Ann Thorac Surg 2006; 82(5): 1842-8.
[http://dx.doi.org/10.1016/j.athoracsur.2006.05.088]

[81]   Marasco SF, Bailey M, McGlade D, *et al.* Effect of donor preservation solution and survival in lung transplantation. J Heart Lung Transplant 2011; 30(4): 414-9.
[http://dx.doi.org/10.1016/j.healun.2010.10.002]

[82]   Gámez P, Córdoba M, Millán I, *et al.* Improvements in lung preservation: 3 years' experience with a low-potassium dextran solution. Arch Bronconeumol 2005; 41(1): 16-9.

[83]   Ganesh JS, Rogers CA, Banner NR, Bonser RS. Audit SGotUCT. Does the method of lung preservation influence outcome after transplantation? An analysis of 681 consecutive procedures. J Thorac Cardiovasc Surg 2007; 134(5): 1313-21.
[http://dx.doi.org/10.1016/j.jtcvs.2007.05.030]

[84]   Hardesty RL, Aeba R, Armitage JM, Kormos RL, Griffith BP. A clinical trial of University of Wisconsin solution for pulmonary preservation. J Thorac Cardiovasc Surg 1993; 105(4): 660-6.

[85]   Müller C, Fürst H, Reichenspurner H, Briegel J, Groh J, Reichart B. Lung procurement by low-potassium dextran and the effect on preservation injury. Munich Lung Transplant Group. Transplantation 1999; 68(8): 1139-43.
[http://dx.doi.org/10.1097/00007890-199910270-00014]

[86]   Rabanal JM, Ibañez AM, Mons R, *et al.* Influence of preservation solution on early lung function (Euro-Collins vs Perfadex). Transplant Proc 2003; 35(5): 1938-9.
[http://dx.doi.org/10.1016/S0041-1345(03)00690-0]

[87]   Strüber M, Wilhelmi M, Harringer W, *et al.* Flush perfusion with low potassium dextran solution improves early graft function in clinical lung transplantation. Eur J Cardiothorac Surg 2001; 19(2): 190-4.
[http://dx.doi.org/10.1016/S1010-7940(00)00631-X]

[88]   Fischer S, Meyer K, Tessmann R, *et al.* Outcome following single vs bilateral lung transplantation in recipients 60 years of age and older. Transplant Proc 2005; 37(2): 1369-70.

[http://dx.doi.org/10.1016/j.transproceed.2004.12.269]

[89]   't Hart NA, van der Plaats A, Moers C, *et al.* Development of the isolated dual perfused rat liver model as an improved reperfusion model for transplantation research. Int J Artif Organs 2006; 29(2): 219-27.
[http://dx.doi.org/10.1177/039139880602900208]

CHAPTER 7

Organ Specific Considerations: Heart

Vincent Nardy[1], **Ahmet Kilic**[2,*] and **Arman Kilic**[3]

[1] *The Ohio State University, Columbus, OH, USA*

[2] *Johns Hopkins University, Baltimore, MD, USA*

[3] *University of Pittsburgh, Pittsburgh, PA, USA*

Abstract: Cardiac allograft evaluation and procurement are integral parts of the multiorgan donation process as cardiac function prior to brain death determination often has a critical impact on multiorgan function. In this chapter, the authors review the basic principles of cardiac assessment as well as maintaining cardiopulmonary function during the period after brain death determination to enhance overall cardiopulmonary as well as abdominal organ perfusion and function. They also review acceptable donor criteria, expanding the donor criteria to enhance organ availability, preservation solution selection and techniques and donor-recipient selection and matching to improve post transplant success.

Keywords: Donor Criteria, Donor-Recipient Matching in Heart Transplantation, Extended Donor Criteria.

INTRODUCTION

While there have been significant advances in the field of cardiac transplant which has allowed for a larger pool of potential recipients, the persistent shortcoming continues to be the lack of adequate available donors. Over the last two decades, the number of transplants being performed in the United States has remained roughly constant at 2,000 – 2,500 per year. This imbalance between supply and demand has placed a lot of pressure on transplant surgeons nationwide to assure appropriate donor selection and allocation. As such, the Centers for Medicare and Medicaid Services (CMS) have raised the standards for individual institutions to assure they continue to meet national mortality and graft survival standards. One of the most influential components of both patient and graft survival is identifying the appropriate donor organ.

---

* **Corresponding author Ahmet Kilic:** Johns Hopkins University, Baltimore, MD, USA; Tel: 4109552800; Fax: 4109553809; Emails: akilic2@jhmi.edu; ahmetkilic@yahoo.com

Robert S.D. Higgins & Juan A. Sanchez (Eds.)

Donor and Recipient Selection

Although most institutions can agree on some basic criteria for discussions on how to select both transplant donors and recipients, there exist significant variations amongst institutions, regions and individual physicians. The work up to place someone on the transplant list is extensive and typically requires a multidisciplinary approach. Patients undergoing evaluation for heart transplantation generally are patients with New York Heart Association Class IV symptoms with heart failure on maximal medical therapy, intractable anginal symptoms refractive to medical or surgical therapy, malignant ventricular arrhythmias, and/or patients not expected to survive more than 2-3 years without a transplant.

Donor evaluation can be overly simplified into quality of the donor followed by suitability for the specific recipient. A reasonable approach is to have a mental checklist as a primary survey to ensure appropriate ABO blood typing, demographics, expected ischemic time, confirmation of brain death, verification of consent to donate, identification of co-morbid conditions (high risk sexual behaviors or substance abuse, mechanism of death, the need for and duration of cardiopulmonary resuscitation). The quality of the donor heart can be evaluated by the history, mechanism of death, cardiac enzymes, electrocardiogram, hemodynamic stability with special attention to pressor or inotrope support, echocardiogram and in selected cases, coronary angiogram. Echocardiogram is the cornerstone of decision making as it can show the function of each ventricle, ejection fraction, septal hypertrophy, diastolic dysfunction, valvular abnormalities and other congenital abnormalities that can negatively impact the success of transplantation. Coronary angiogram is typically reserved for patients > 50 years of age, those with wall motion abnormalities, co-morbid conditions for ischemia and those with suspicion for myocardial infarction or embolus on cardiac enzymes or electrocardiogram. Finally, visual and manual inspection for external injuries or anomalies by the surgeon is performed to confirm the final acceptability of the organ at the time of procurement. In 2002, a consensus conference came up with The Crystal City Guidelines and developed a summary algorithm to aid in the selection and management of potential donors (Table **7.1**).

Of all the criteria used while evaluating donor-recipient compatibility, there are a few that are particularly noteworthy. Age of the donor plays an essential role when determining if the donor heart will meet the long-term needs of the recipient. In earlier more conservative days, most centers limited their criteria to donors under the age of 35. However, due to the imbalance between supply and demand, most centers have expanded their criteria to include donors into their fifth decade. In an attempt to increase the donor pool further, some have advocated to include patients into their sixth decade. However, after reviewing data from the National Transplant Cardiologist Database of 10,000 heart recipients, we have evidence demonstrating higher risk for early mortality when the donor was over the age of 60 [1]. Naturally, older donors have a higher prevalence for coronary artery disease. This is significant because older donors and donors with coronary artery disease have been correlated to have coronary allograft vasculopathy [2]. For this reason, angiogram should be at least considered for donors > 40 years of age or with significant risk factors (hypertension, diabetes, hyperlipidemia, or smoker). Two other important factors when evaluating compatibility are both the gender and size (height/weight/BMI) of the donor and recipient. Gender mismatching is clinically more pronounced when a female donor heart is placed in a male recipient. This particular scenario is associated with both a higher frequency and severity of graft rejection [3]. When looking at size mismatching, using BMI or height may offer a more precise estimate than just weight alone. Similar to age mismatching, size mismatch, both undersizing and oversizing, portends worse outcomes. Therefore, accepted clinical practice of having donor-recipient weight or BMI within 20-30% of each other has been shown to offer the best outcomes [4].

One potential method of expanding the donor pool is to include donors that are considered "suboptimal." However, it comes as no surprise, by accepting organs from donors that already have a precarious clinical state, the risk for adverse outcomes is present. Sweeny *et al.,* defined high risk donors as having any of the following: age > 50, sepsis, required CPR > 3 minutes, ischemic time > 5hrs, recreational drug use, weight > 20% less than recipient, and inotropic support > 10-20 µg/kg/min. When they compared the hospital mortality (30 day), 12 month survival, and left ventricular function between high risk donors and non-high risk donors, there was no statistical significance [1]. This contrasts the findings of group from the Cardiac Transplant Research Database which investigated the impact of donor-related predictors of postoperative morbidity and mortality. They reviewed data from multiple institutions and specifically tried to focus on using an "extended donor criteria." They found risk factors for death included older donor age, smaller donor body surface area, higher donor inotropic support, donors with diabetes, longer ischemic time, and donors with diffuse wall motion abnormalities on echocardiography. Specifically, they found donors over the age of 50 years and Dopamine (or Dobutamine) support greater than 20 µg/kg/min, had a significant increase in their overall 30-day mortality of 11% and 12%, respectfully [5]. The solution to solving the imbalance between supply and demand is certainly complex and will require further research and technological advances from both ends. It entails strict and careful donor section along with compulsive attention to detail regarding surgical technique during procurement and re-implantation. This is in conjunction with broadening our understanding of transplant immunology for developing novel therapeutic treatments and making refinements to produce smaller, safer, and more efficient mechanical support devices.

Table 7.1. Guidelines for the Management of Heart Donors. The Crystal City Guidelines for an algorithm for the management of potential heart donors [12]. CVP = central venous pressures, HCT = hematocrit, Hgb = hemoglobin, MAP = mean arterial pressure, LVEF = left ventricular ejection fraction; T3 = triiodothyronine, SVR = systemic vascalar resistance, BG = blood glucose, PCWP = pulmonary capillary wedge pressure. (Circulation 2002; 109:836-41).

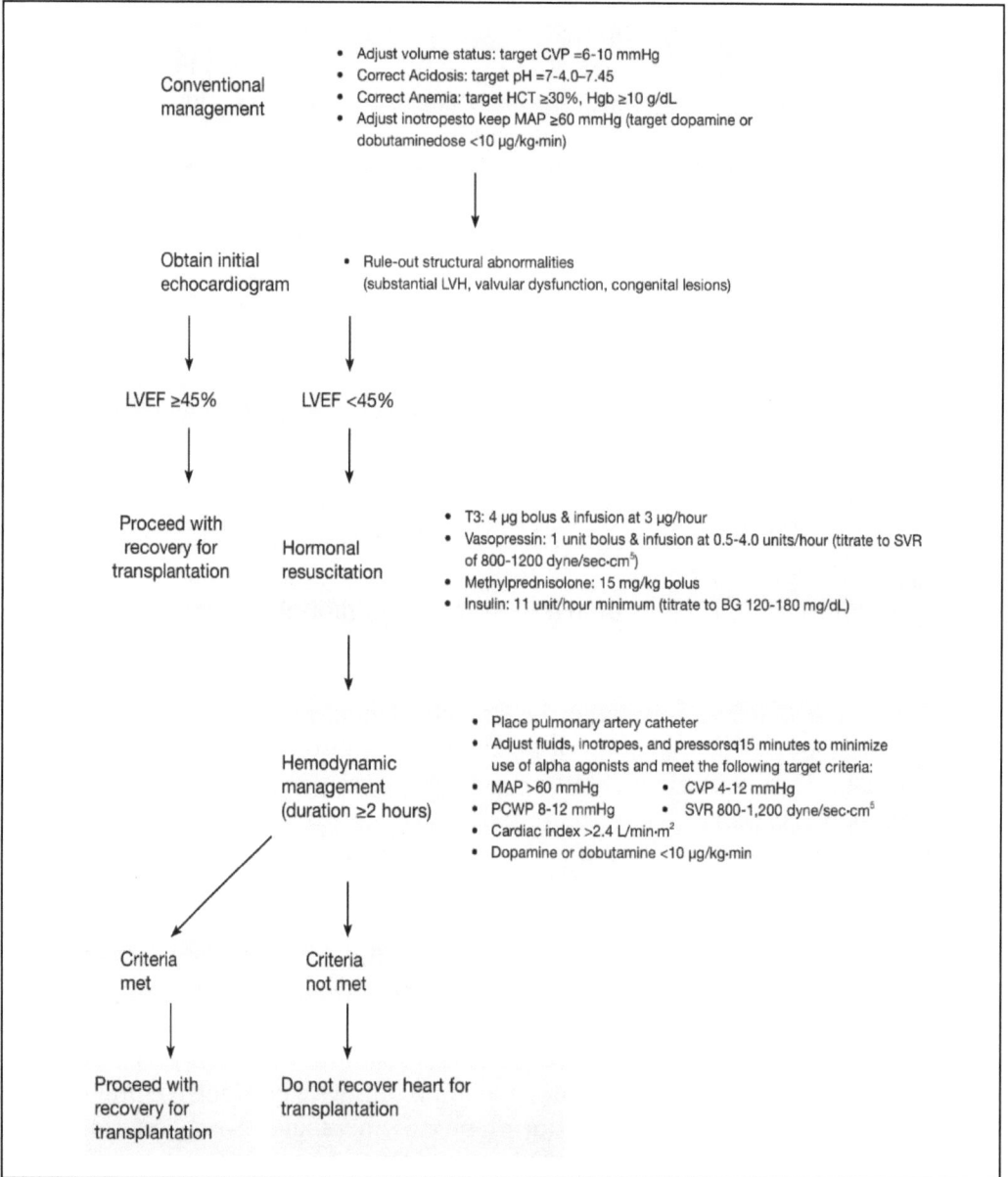

Conventional management
- Adjust volume status: target CVP =6-10 mmHg
- Correct Acidosis: target pH =7-4.0–7.45
- Correct Anemia: target HCT ≥30%, Hgb ≥10 g/dL
- Adjust inotropes to keep MAP ≥60 mmHg (target dopamine or dobutamine dose <10 µg/kg·min)

Obtain initial echocardiogram
- Rule-out structural abnormalities (substantial LVH, valvular dysfunction, congenital lesions)

LVEF ≥45%   **LVEF <45%**

Proceed with recovery for transplantation

Hormonal resuscitation
- T3: 4 µg bolus & infusion at 3 µg/hour
- Vasopressin: 1 unit bolus & infusion at 0.5-4.0 units/hour (titrate to SVR of 800-1200 dyne/sec·cm^5)
- Methylprednisolone: 15 mg/kg bolus
- Insulin: 11 unit/hour minimum (titrate to BG 120-180 mg/dL)

Hemodynamic management (duration ≥2 hours)
- Place pulmonary artery catheter
- Adjust fluids, inotropes, and pressors q15 minutes to minimize use of alpha agonists and meet the following target criteria:
- MAP >60 mmHg   CVP 4-12 mmHg
- PCWP 8-12 mmHg   SVR 800-1,200 dyne/sec·cm^5
- Cardiac index >2.4 L/min·m^2
- Dopamine or dobutamine <10 µg/kg·min

Criteria met   **Criteria not met**

Proceed with recovery for transplantation   **Do not recover heart for transplantation**

Patient Management and Preservation Strategies

Prior to explantation of the organs, it is imperative to maintain donor homeostasis as much as possible. The pathophysiologic changes that accompany brain death can be complex with erratic fluctuations in clinical status. The goals of care for a transplant donor are not much different than those of any other critically ill patient. Specific goals include maintaining a mean arterial pressure (MAP) greater than 60 mm Hg (or systolic blood pressure greater than 90 mm Hg), urine output greater than 30 mL but less than 300 mL per hour, maintaining normal temperature and pH, and finally maintaining optimal cardiopulmonary function to allow for adequate tissue oxygenation, ventilation, and perfusion.

One of the greatest advances in transplantation was the use and understanding of tissue preservation. There are four basic preservation strategies that can be used individually or in combination with each other. These include hypothermia alone, hypothermic perfusate (cardioplegia), donor cooling via cardiopulmonary bypass, and continuous perfusion (autoperfusion). While bypass can rapidly achieve whole-body hypothermia and improve preservation, it requires axillary staff for technical support and may increase risk of organ injury during dissection and cannulation. Thus, it is rarely used in the United States. The most widely used technique is topical cold storage with a cold cardioplegia perfusate. Some of the more common cardioplegia solutions utilized in the United States are the Stanford solution and the modified EuroCollins solution [6]. Another solution developed by Dr. Belzer at the University of Wisconsin, has been shown to increase the preservation time from 6 hours to 24 hours in some solid organs [7]. Its composition includes: low-molecular-weight molecules; albumin; nucleotide precursors adenosine and ribose; antioxidants like glutathione and allopurinol; and metabolic substrates such as glycogen, fructose, and free fatty acids. Therefore, it helps to suppress cellular edema and preserve metabolism by stabilizing the cellular environment [8].

Procurement Technique

Retrieval of the heart is usually performed as part of a multi-organ procurement and typically in conjunction with one or more transplant teams. Ongoing communication between various teams is critical in preventing prolonged ischemic times. This includes discussions on start times based on transportation and travel. Just as important is communication with the recipient team, as redo sternotomy and LVAD explantation are becoming much more frequent and can require additional time. The heart is accessed through a median sternotomy followed by opening the pericardium longitudinally (Fig. **7.1**). The heart is carefully inspected for any signs of trauma, infarction, congenital anomalies, and overall right and left ventricular function. The coronary arteries should also be palpated to evaluate for coronary artery disease or anatomic variations. It is at this point the final decision to accept or decline the heart for transplant can be made. The ascending aorta is carefully dissected off the pulmonary artery and encircled with umbilical tape. The inferior vena cava (IVC) and superior vena cava (SVC) are mobilized from the diaphragm up until the SVC-azygos vein junction is identified. The IVC is then encircled with umbilical tape, the SVC with a silk tie, and the azygos vein doubly ligated with a silk time but not transecting it. Once the abdominal team and recipient team are ready, 30,000 units of intravenous heparin is given to the donor and allowed to circulate for three minutes. Systemic heparinization is the key to prevent microvascular thrombosis and heparin must be given with enough time for it to circulate prior to the cross clamp being applied.

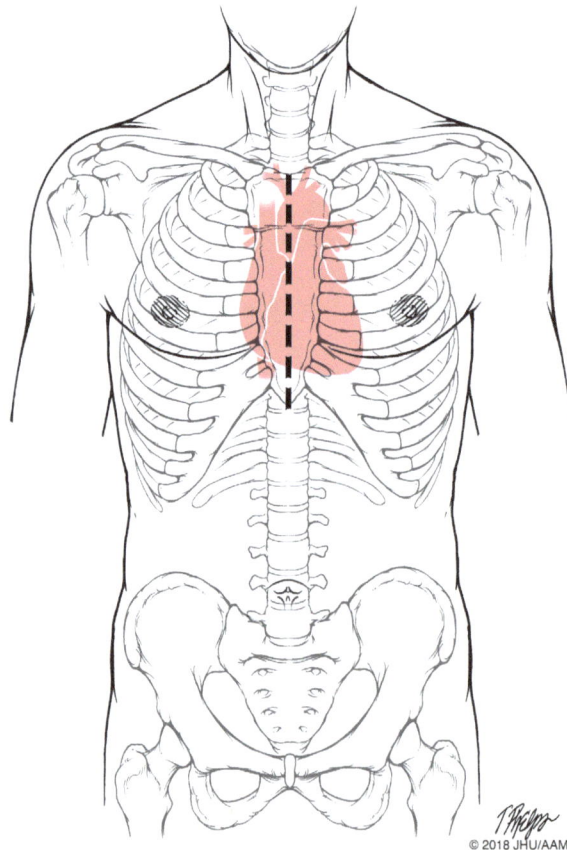

Fig. (7.1). Median Sternotomy for heart procurement: The heart is accessed through a median sternotomy followed by opening the pericardium longitudinally. Medical Illustrations© 2018 Tim Phelps, MS, FAMI, Johns Hopkins University.

During this time, a cardioplegia needle is inserted into the ascending aorta and connected to a pressurized bag containing the crystalloid preservation solution. It is important at this juncture to ensure all central venous lines are pulled back from the SVC. The SVC is then snared tightly to limit venous return to the heart. The right heart is decompressed, and the donor is exsanguinated by incising the (IVC) at the diaphragm (Fig. **7.2**). A pitfall for this procedure can occur at this point if there is poor communication between amongst the various procurement teams. It is critical to confirm sufficient length on the SVC and IVC cuffs, as these will be needed later for bicaval anastomoses during recipient implantation. Blood and perfusate from the liver will drain into the right pleural cavity, and suction should be available to keep the field clear. The aortic clamp is then placed as high on the aorta as possible once the heart begins to empty. The left side of the heart is allowed to decompress by incising either the left or right inferior pulmonary vein and if left ventricular distension persists, incising the left atrial appendage can be done to also help with decompression. Avoidance of left ventricular distension is critical in minimizing myocardial stress and regionalized hypoxemia and acidosis prior to procurement. Expeditious troubleshooting ensuring appropriate control of inflow to the heart (SVC and IVC) as well as appropriate excision of left atrial appendage, left atrium and/or pulmonary veins to provide LV venting is crucial to success of the procurement procedure (Fig. **7.3**).

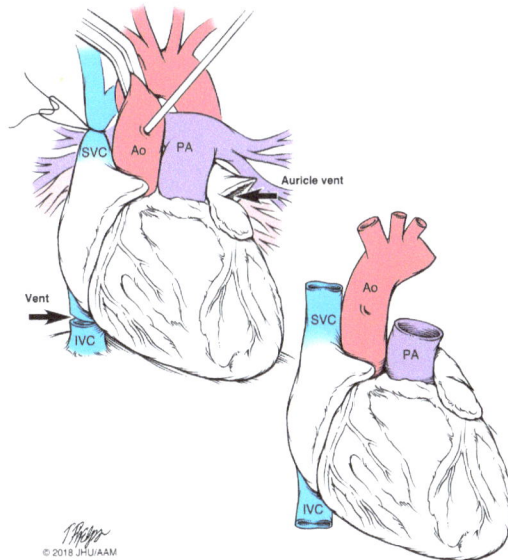

Fig. (7.2). Administration of cardioplegic preservation solution following clamping of the ascending aorta. The right heart is vented by an incision in the inferior vena cava. The left heart is vented trhough the left atrial appendage. Medical Illustrations© 2018 Tim Phelps, MS, FAMI, Johns Hopkins University.

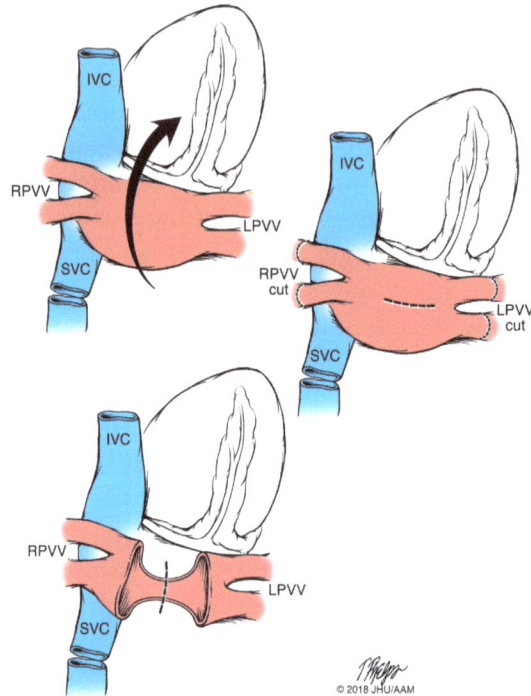

Fig. (7.3). During the donor procurement procedure of the heart, if the lungs are not being utilized the pulmonary veins can be divided at the level of the pericardial reflection to maximize cuff lengths. Conversely, if the lungs are to be utilized for transplantation, the left atrial cuff remains attached to the set of pulmonary veins with the line of incision as shown. Medical Illustrations© 2018 Tim Phelps, MS, FAMI, Johns Hopkins University.

The cardioplegia solution is then rapidly infused into the aorta leading to diastolic arrest. Topical hypothermia is achieved with several liters of ice cold slush to assist with preservation. Once the cardioplegia solution has finished infusing, heart is excised. It is worth noting that this part of the procedure is the foundation for the whole transplant. It is imperative to move quickly but deliberately as any mistake at this juncture can jeopardize the organ. The aorta is divided high at the cross clamp and the heart retracted cephalad. It is increasingly more common that the heart transplant recipient is a redo sternotomy with prior aortic manipulation and taking the aorta at the level past the great vessels should be the common practice during procurement. Finally, the pulmonary veins, the SVC, the IVC are divided along with the pulmonary artery, which is divided near the bifurcation. As mentioned previously, obtaining adequate length on these structures is extremely important. For example, having inappropriate length on the IVC can lead to impingement of the coronary sinus. Similar pitfalls are true for the SVC and pulmonary artery. Not enough length on either can lead to undue stress on the donor-recipient anastomosis and inappropriate pulmonary arterial length will need augmentation using either autologous or bovine pericardium. For this reason, a piece of pericardium should also be harvested in the event any reconstruction is needed. The heart is then immediately placed in a sterile bag of saline cooled to 4°C which is then placed into one to two other bags filled with saline. It is then safely packaged on ice for transport. It should be noted that there are a few variations in technique when excising the heart that are dependent upon the lungs being harvested simultaneously. If the lungs are not being harvested, division of the pulmonary veins can take place at the pericardial reflection. Conversely, if the lungs are being used to transplant, a midatrial incision can be made to create a left atrial cuff and a separate pulmonary venous cuff. Lastly, the heart and lungs can be explanted *en-bloc* and separated out on the back table [9, 10].

FUTURE DIRECTIONS

Currently in organ procurement, preservation and minimization of harm is the key concept with the ultimate goal to narrow the gap between donor-recipient supply and demand. Akin to kidney transplantation and more recently lung transplantation, the future direction of heart transplantation will be the repair of hearts utilizing *ex vivo* methods of repairing organs that were once deemed unsuitable or "marginal". The PROCEED II trial prospectively randomized 130 patients at multiple institutions in the United States and Europe to *ex-vivo* perfusion prior to implantation versus standard cold storage. They were able to demonstrate similar patient and graft survival at 30 days using both methods [11]. Similarly, a case series out of Australia used *ex-vivo* for three hearts with distant procurements donated after circulatory death (DCD). Despite two patients needing temporary mechanical support postoperatively, all three had a good recovery by one week with one of the patients still doing well at 176 days post-transplant [12]. Despite these encouraging results, there still needs to be more basic science and long term clinical research before utilizing *ex-vivo* perfusion systems routinely.

CONSENT FOR PUBLICATION

Not applicable.

CONFLICT OF INTEREST

The author declares no conflict of interest, financial or otherwise.

ACKNOWLEDGEMENTS

Declared none.

REFERENCES

[1]   Sweeney MS, Lammermeier DE, Frazier OH, Burnett CM, Haupt HM, Duncan JM. Extension of donor criteria in cardiac transplantation: surgical risk versus supply-side economics. Ann Thorac Surg 1990; 50(1): 7-10.
[http://dx.doi.org/10.1016/0003-4975(90)90071-D] [PMID: 2369232]

[2]   Gao HZ, Hunt SA, Alderman EL, Liang D, Yeung AC, Schroeder JS. Relation of donor age and preexisting coronary artery disease on angiography and intracoronary ultrasound to later development of accelerated allograft coronary artery disease. J Am Coll Cardiol 1997; 29(3): 623-9.
[http://dx.doi.org/10.1016/S0735-1097(96)00521-9] [PMID: 9060902]

[3]   Welp H, Spieker T, Erren M, Scheld HH, Baba HA, Stypmann J. Sex mismatch in heart transplantation is associated with increased number of severe rejection episodes and shorter long-term survival. Transplant Proc 2009; 41(6): 2579-84.
[http://dx.doi.org/10.1016/j.transproceed.2009.06.098] [PMID: 19715978]

[4]   Blackbourne LH, Tribble CG, Langenburg SE, *et al.* Successful use of undersized donors for orthotopic heart transplantation--with a caveat. Ann Thorac Surg 1994; 57(6): 1472-5.
[http://dx.doi.org/10.1016/0003-4975(94)90103-1] [PMID: 8010789]

[5]   Young JB, Naftel DC, Bourge RC, *et al.* Matching the heart donor and heart transplant recipient. Clues for successful expansion of the donor pool: a multivariable, multiinstitutional report. J Heart Lung Transplant 1994; 13(3): 353-64.
[PMID: 8061010]

[6]   Baldwin JC, Frist WH, Starkey TD, *et al.* Distant graft procurement for combined heart and lung transplantation using pulmonary artery flush and simple topical hypothermia for graft preservation. Ann Thorac Surg 1987; 43(6): 670-3.
[http://dx.doi.org/10.1016/S0003-4975(10)60249-4] [PMID: 3109339]

[7]   Belzer FO, Southard JH. Principles of solid-organ preservation by cold storage. Transplantation 1988; 45(4): 673-6.
[http://dx.doi.org/10.1097/00007890-198804000-00001] [PMID: 3282347]

[8]   Aziz S, Tada Y, Jaffery S, *et al.* University of Wisconsin solution provides superior myocardial preservation compared with Stanford cardioplegic solution. J Heart Lung Transplant 1994; 13(6): 1099-108.
[PMID: 7865517]

[9]   Chiu P, Robbins R, Ha R. Heart Transplant.Sabiston and Spencer Surgery of the Chest. 9th ed. Philadelphia: Elsevier 2016; pp. 1736-9.

[10]   Pasque MK. Standardizing thoracic organ procurement for transplantation. J Thorac Cardiovasc Surg 2010; 139(1): 13-7.
[http://dx.doi.org/10.1016/j.jtcvs.2009.09.015] [PMID: 20106357]

[11]   Ardehali A, Esmailian F, Deng M, *et al.* Ex-vivo perfusion of donor hearts for human heart transplantation (PROCEED II): a prospective, open-label, multicentre, randomised non-inferiority trial. Lancet 2015; 385(9987): 2577-84.
[http://dx.doi.org/10.1016/S0140-6736(15)60261-6] [PMID: 25888086]

[12]   Dhital KK, Iyer A, Connellan M, *et al.* Adult heart transplantation with distant procurement and *ex-vivo* preservation of donor hearts after circulatory death: a case series. Lancet 2015; 385(9987): 2585-91.
[http://dx.doi.org/10.1016/S0140-6736(15)60038-1] [PMID: 25888085]

CHAPTER 8

Organ Specific Considerations: Lung

Jinny Ha, Stephen Broderick and **Errol Bush**[*]

Johns Hopkins University School of Medicine, Baltimore, MD, USA

Abstract: Donor lung assessment has evolved significantly as experience grows in the field of cardiopulmonary transplantation and organ donors are more actively managed with consideration of their pulmonary function. This chapter evaluates the current criteria employed in many centers evaluating traditional assessments of oxygenation and ventilation to avoid early graft dysfunction secondary to ischemia-reperfusion injury using modern ventilator and preservation fluids and techniques.

Keywords: Expanded Criteria Lung Donors, Donor-Recipient Matching, Lung Donation Standard Criteria, Lung Transplantation- Primary Graft Dysfunction.

INTRODUCTION

Much progress has been made since the first lung transplant performed nearly thirty years ago. Lung transplantation remains a mainstay treatment for end stage respiratory pathologies, but remains an imperfect therapeutic option. A greater understanding of the impact of donor characteristics on the recipient outcomes has allowed us to refine and expand the donor pool available. This chapter will present and review the pertinent data supporting current donor selection criteria as well as step-by-step description of a standard double lung en-bloc recovery for transplantation.

Donor Criteria

Ischemia-reperfusion injury remains a significant cause of early morbidity and mortality after lung transplantation. Insults that occur before lung donation and during preservation and implantation can contribute to the development of primary graft dysfunction (PGD) [1]. PGD has been previously reported to have an incidence of 10-30%, while a current era study by Diamond *et al* demonstrates an incidence of approximately 17% 2-3 days following transplant, which translated into a 3-5x increased risk of short-term mortality [2]. Both donor

[*] **Corresponding author Errol Bush:** Johns Hopkins University School of Medicine, Baltimore, MD, USA; Tel: 410-614-3891; Fax: 443-267-0188; Email: errol.bush@jhmi.edu

Robert S.D. Higgins & Juan A. Sanchez (Eds.)

characteristics and acquired donor factors that occur around the period of donation have been shown to impact recipient outcomes and the incidence of PGD [3]. Therefore, careful donor selection, management, and organ recovery are important for achieving good short-term outcomes.

The "standard criteria" for selecting the ideal lung donor were developed from the early initial lung transplant successes and experiences from small institutional studies [4] (Table **8.1**). Transplant centers vary in the donor selection criteria and have advocated the use of extended criteria donors to increase the pool of available donors. The rationale and impact of individual factors will be reviewed here.

Table 8.1. Ideal lung donor criteria.

Ideal Lung Donor Criteria
Age <55 years old
Clear serial chest x-ray
Normal gas exchange (PaO_2:FiO_2 ratio >350)
Less than 5 ventilation days
Absence of organism on sputum gram stain
Clear bronchoscopy
Ischemia time <4 hours
Tobacco history < 20 pack-years
ABO compatibility
Appropriate size match with prospective recipient

Age

The age of donors accepted for transplantation has steadily increased. However, a recent review of the United Network for Organ Sharing (UNOS) database demonstrated that <1% of donors were > 65 years of age and <10% of donors were >55 years of age [8]. Older reviews of the International Society of Heart and Lung Transplantation (ISHLT) data have demonstrated worse early and late survival outcomes with the use of older donors [5 - 7]. Later studies using donors with age >50 showed similar long- and short-term outcomes in recipients who received transplants from younger donors [7, 8]. In a retrospective review of the UNOS data, 1- and 3- year mortality for donors 55-64 were similar for standard criteria donors; however, donors >65 had worse early and intermediate survival outcomes [9]. In the current era, Holley *et al* recently demonstrated in a single institution study, no significant difference in PGD, survival or chronic allograft dysfunction in recipients receiving organs from older donors, but there was perioperative increase in resource utilization [10]. Katsnelson *et al* further demonstrated, using the UNOS database, no significant differences in short- nor long-term outcomes utilizing older donors when donor age was within 10 years of the recipient [11]. Based on the current available evidence, older donor lungs should be carefully considered for transplantation and should not be rejected based on age alone.

Smoking History

A retrospective review of UNOS data from 2005 to 2011, the incidence of bronchiolitis obliterans syndrome (BOS) and median survival of recipients of grafts from donors with heavy smoking history (>20 pack years) were not worse than non-smoking donors [12]. Another study found that donor smoking history negatively impacted early outcomes in a dose-dependent manner, but there was no significant effect on long-term outcomes [13]. A donor history of tobacco use should not be excluded from transplantation; however, smoking increases the risk for transplanting undetected malignancies. Chest x-rays and CT scans must be carefully reviewed to identify any potential malignancies. The authors encourage a CT scan of the chest for all donors with a smoking history > 20py that is carefully reviewed by an attending radiologist and the surgical team prior to recovery to evaluate for any tobacco related changes and suspicious nodules or undiagnosed malignancies.

ABO Compatibility

There is no significant disadvantage to use ABO-compatible compared to ABO-identical donors. A study comparing ABO-identical to ABO-compatible donors did not identify any significant difference in one-year survival or incidence in acute or chronic rejection [14]. Despite these findings, Taghavi *et al* reviewed the UNOS database and also found that there is no difference in short and long-term outcomes, however still only 8% of adult lung transplants are performed with ABO compatible donors [15]. ABO incompatibility still remains an absolute contraindication to donor acceptability in the adult recipient population.

Size Criteria

Based on a review of a few older studies, there are no clinical or functional adverse outcomes after double-lung transplant when the donor predicted total lung capacity (TLC) is between 75 to 125% of the recipient total lung capacity [16]. Size matching is typically done based on donor and recipient height and the predicted total lung capacity. Sizing may be further tailored based on the recipient's lung disease. Larger lungs can be used in recipients with hyperinflated conditions, such as COPD or cystic fibrosis. Restrictive lung disease causes the chest wall to shrink. In these cases, donor lungs from smaller donors would be acceptable. In cases of significantly oversized organs, lung reduction in the form of wedge resection or lobectomies can be performed at the time of transplantation to better accommodate the recipient's chest cavity. It should be noted that a higher predicted TLC ratio has been associated with at least improved short-term survival, especially in double lung transplant recipients, suggesting judicious use of techniques to downsize oversized lungs [17].

Graft Ischemia

Most transplant centers accept an ischemia time of approximately 4 to 6 hours, however, the upper limit of graft ischemia time is unknown. The data regarding the impact on ischemia time and survival is conflicting. A multivariate analysis of UNOS registry data demonstrated an increase in 1-year mortality in patients with graft ischemia times >7 hours when combined with older donor age (>55 years). In this study, however, an ischemia time of > 7 hours alone did not increase recipient mortality [18]. Smaller single center studies report a worse survival with graft ischemia times >5 hours [19, 20]. While another retrospective analysis of UNOS registry data of lung transplant recipients between 2000-2005 showed that ischemia times >6 hours was not an independent predictor of mortality [21]. In the current era, no association was found between prolonged total graft ischemia times (TGIT) and primary graft failure or survival following lung transplantation, even upwards to 12 hours TGIT [22]. While it appears that carefully selected donors can be safely utilized even when predicted TGIT will be prolonged and the upper limit of acceptable TGIT still remains elusive, it is still prudent to minimize TGIT when logistically possible.

Radiographic Findings

Donors undergo multiple chest radiographs and CT scans prior to recovery, which provide information regarding the presence of infiltrates, masses, pulmonary edema or contusions. There is, however, a significant amount of inter-observer variability when interpreting these images to determine donor suitability [23]. There are no firm guidelines established regarding the utilization of donors with abnormal chest x-rays. Infiltrates or opacities on a chest x-ray, in conjunction with fever and leukocytosis are highly suspicious of pneumonia. These clinical findings should be further investigated with bronchoscopy to evaluate the extent and characteristics of pulmonary secretions.

Bronchoscopy and Gram Stain

Bronchoscopic evaluation of donor lungs is an imperative part of the donor selection process. The donor organs must be inspected for persistent purulent secretions, evidence of aspiration, and identification of anatomical abnormalities or injuries that would preclude transplantation. Aspiration is a common event in donation after brain death donors, owing mostly to common mechanisms of injury and the often emergent intubation process. Lungs with gross evidence of diffuse inflammation, infection or aspiration are typically not accepted for transplantation. Bronchial washings or tracheal aspirates are frequently found to have positive gram stains. Studies have shown that positive gram stains do not translate to the development of subsequent pneumonia post-transplantation or need for prolonged mechanical ventilation [24]. One study demonstrated that despite an incidence of 52% of donor infections being evident, only 8% of donor to recipient transmission of infection occurred [25]. Transmissions of infections can be mitigated with the use of preemptive antibiotic regimens in donors prior to the recovery procedure and appropriate prophylactic antibiotic regimens in recipients pre-operatively.

Gas Exchange

The arterial partial pressure of oxygen (PaO_2) to FiO_2 ratio is important in assessing the gas exchange of donor lungs. The ideal PaO_2/FiO_2 of >300 mmHg should be achieved on FiO_2 = 1.0, PEEP = 5 cm H_2O. Causes for lower oxygenation such as atelectasis and mucous plugging are reversible. Aggressive recruitment maneuvers should be performed to improve gas exchange. Exclusion of unilateral lesions may improve oxygenation. Taking individual pulmonary vein gas samples may provide additional information when considering single lung transplants.

Donor lungs should have normal PCO_2 levels (35 to 45 mmHg). Derangements of gas exchange resulting in hypercapnia in a donor may signify underlying pathologies that are acute or chronic in nature. More acute processes that contribute to elevated PCO_2 levels include edema, infections, and acute lung injury. In older donors or donors with significant smoking history, hypercapnia suggests more advanced COPD, asthma or bronchiectasis.

Techniques for Donor Lung Extraction

Initial On-site Evaluation of the Donor Organ

Upon arrival to the donor hospital or facility, the donor and recipient ABO compatibility, brain death evaluation and declaration, and consent for donation are confirmed. Any other pertinent history of the donor, such as the mechanism of injury, past medical history and donor serologies, is reviewed. The recovery team should evaluate any pertinent imaging. A fiber optic bronchoscopy should be performed to identify any anatomic abnormalities and to ensure there are no significant secretions. During bronchoscopy, secretions should clear easily and should not reaccumulate. Arterial blood gases should be obtained with the FiO_2 at 100% with a PEEP of 5. Any abnormalities or concerns are quickly reported back to the recipient team.

Positioning

The donor is placed supine with both arms tucked. Central lines in the neck or chest should be excluded from the prepped surgical field. The skin should be prepped from the chin to the pubis for recovery of both thoracic and abdominal organs.

Initial Gross Evaluation of the Donor Lungs

Prior to incision, most OPOs perform a moment of silence. This time is a period that should be utilized to reflect upon the sacrifice and gift that the donor and donor family are about to bestow upon potentially multiple recipients. It is also during this time, that the recovering surgeons should remember that the recovery operation can result in donor instability and organ injury, therefore each step should be performed utilizing safe techniques and without haste. Sometimes the full intended dissection is not safe to perform prior to cross-clamp and the recovery surgeon must be vigilant enough to recognize this risk.

The heart and lungs are exposed *via* a median sternotomy with extension to a midline laparotomy to the pubis for abdominal organ recovery (Fig. **8.1**). Both pleural spaces are opened with cautery down to the level of the diaphragm and up to the pedicle of the intrathoracic mammary vessels. Care must be taken not to inadvertently injure the lungs. Each lung is delivered out of the pleural space for a gross inspection. Aggressive evisceration of the lungs may cause injury to the hilar structure or lead to hemodynamic instability. Lung evisceration is usually better tolerated if performed before the pericardium is open, but the order of thoracic organ evaluation must be carefully coordinated with the heart team, if there is a separate team. During the inspection, any areas of contusion or consolidation should be noted. Additionally, edema and compliance of lungs should be evaluated. Atelectatic segments of lung should be recruited gently with hand ventilation to pressures of starting at 20 up to 40 cm H_2O. Hyperinflation of the lungs during this maneuver should be avoided. Once the donor lungs are considered acceptable for transplantation, the recipient implant team is notified. An estimate of the donor cross-clamp time is relayed.

Donor Lung Dissection

Pericardial retraction sutures are placed to provide exposure to the great vessels as well as maintaining access to bilateral pleural spaces. Some center recover protocols reserve the vascular and airway dissection until after cross-clamp to avoid potential injury and induced instability. The authors prefer to carefully perform the dissection prior to cross-clamp while the vascular planes are more readily identified and protected while perfused. Based on the experience and comfort level of the recovery surgeon, the particular technique should be chosen. The dissection begins with the mobilization of the superior vena cava (SVC). The attachments between the SVC and the right pulmonary artery should be divided. The SVC should be dissected up the innominate vein and down to the right atrium. The azygous vein should also be identified. A heavy silk suture tie is passed around the SVC below the level of the azygous vein. Dissection on top of the right main pulmonary artery is continued under the aorta, separating the posterior aspect of the aorta from the right pulmonary artery. The aorta is then dissected free from the main pulmonary artery. Careful, dissection of Sondergaard's inter-atrial groove is done sharply to provide an adequate left atrial cuff.

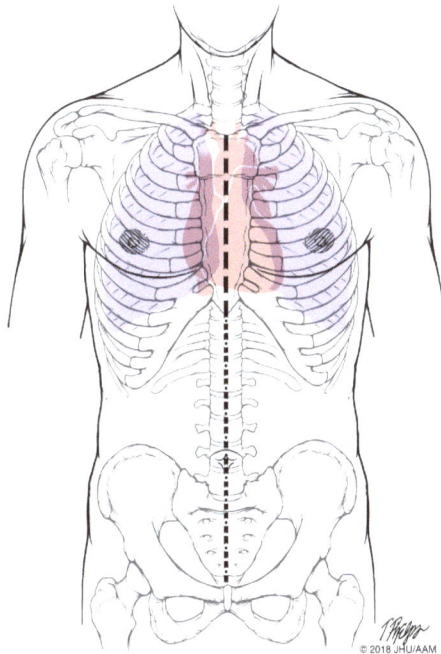

Fig. (8.1). The heart and lungs are exposed *via* a median sternotomy with extension to a midline laparotomy to the pubis for abdominal organ recovery. Medical Illustrations© 2018 Tim Phelps, MS, FAMI, Johns Hopkins University.

Once all recovery teams are ready for cannulation, the donor is heparinized (typically 500 IU/kg, but OPO protocols vary). A 4-0 prolene mattress or purse string cannulation stitch is placed at least 1.5 cm from the pulmonary valve in the distal main pulmonary artery. A large-bore pulmonary artery cannula is placed through a stab incision (Fig. **8.2**). Careful attention is needed to ensure that the pulmonary plegia cannula is directed equally towards the pulmonary artery bifurcation. Alternatively, the cannula is placed in a retrograde fashion towards a competent pulmonary valve to provide equal distribution. The cannula is then secured with a Rummel tourniquet. Prostaglandin E_1 (PGE_1) is administered directly into the pulmonary trunk adjacent to the pulmonary artery cannula, immediately prior to cross-clamp as administration will cause profound hypotension mandating progressing with organ recovery. After the bolus of PGE_1, the SVC is ligated. The left atrial appendage tip is transected to vent the left side of the heart. Next, the IVC is partially transected to further decompress the heart. This is important because it prevents left ventricular distention when cross-clamping the aorta if the heart is also being procured. The aorta is cross-clamped to prevent bronchial artery perfusion. Perfusion with Perfadex preservation solution is given *via* gravity drainage. Topical cold saline is used to bathe the lungs. A total of 2 to 3 L of perfusate is instilled in an antegrade fashion. Ventilation of the lungs should continue during the administration of preservation to promote equal distribution of the perfusate. The procuring surgeon should be vigilant of the effluent from the left atrial appendage, which should run clear if it's adequately perfused.

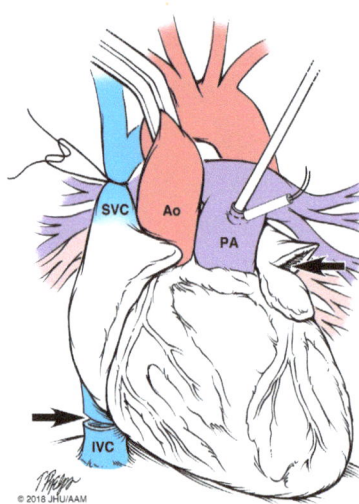

Fig. (8.2). A large-bore pulmonary artery cannula is placed through a stab incision. Medical Illustrations© 2018 Tim Phelps, MS, FAMI, Johns Hopkins University.

Donor Lung Excision

After adequate infusion of preservation solution, the cardiectomy is started. The apex of the heart is lifted up towards the head and the transection of the IVC is completed with favorable cuffs allotted for the heart and liver teams. The left atriotomy is started between the inferior pulmonary veins and the atrioventricular groove. This is continued circumferentially. The left atriotomy is completed from inside the left atrium, while visualizing the four pulmonary vein orifices. The SVC is divided below the silk ligature. The aorta is divided proximal to the cross-clamp. The cannulation site of the main PA is further extended to complete the transection of the main PA. After the heart has been removed from the field, retrograde perfusion with cold Perfadex solution is given with an inflated foley catheter. Each pulmonary vein is individually flushed with approximately 250 mL of perfusate. Return of clear perfusate from the ipsilateral pulmonary artery ensures adequate distribution of the preservation solution. Retrograde perfusion also facilitates clearing of pulmonary emboli.

After the completions of the retrograde flush, the inferior pulmonary ligaments are divided and the mobilization of the posterior mediastinal attachments is completed. The division of the remaining posterior attachments is started inferiorly towards the trachea in the plane anterior to the esophagus. The trachea is bluntly dissected for several centimeters above the carina. A final recruitment maneuver is performed to eradicate residual atelectasis and the lungs are left slightly inflated as the endotracheal tube is withdrawn above the staple line. The trachea is divided in above two fires of the TA-30 stapler. A third staple line can be left on the remnant trachea to avoid further thoracic cavity contamination during the rest of the recovery procedure (Fig. **8.3**).

One variation of this portion of the procedure, performed by some transplant centers, is taking the lung enbloc with the esophagus to minimize devascularization of the airway during the posterior mobilization. After the heart has been removed, one can mobilize and divide the proximal and distal esophagus with a GIA stapler to take the esophagus enbloc with the lungs. All tissue posterior to the esophagus is divided to separate it from the thoracic spine.

The double lung block is placed in a sterile bag filled with cold Perfadex solution. The lungs need to be examined for any surgical injuries or pathologic abnormalities. The first bag is placed in a second bag containing ice slush, followed by a third bag for transport in either an iced cooler or box. The successful recovery of the donor lungs and estimated time of travel is communicated to the implant team.

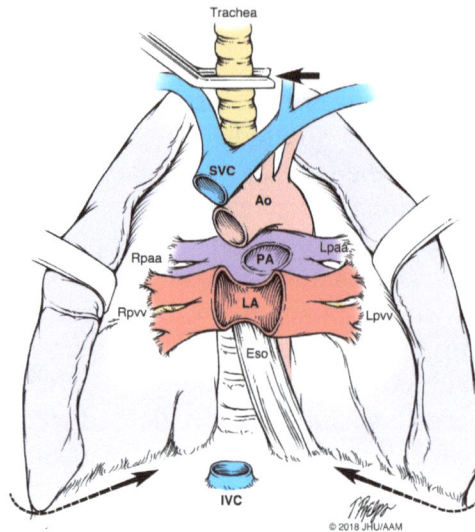

Fig. (8.3). A third staple line can be left on the remnant trachea to avoid further thoracic cavity contamination during the rest of the recovery procedure. Medical Illustrations© 2018 Tim Phelps, MS, FAMI, Johns Hopkins University.

CONCLUSIONS AND FUTURE DIRECTIONS

Despite the major advances in organ preservations and immunosuppression, the goal of achieving long term lung allograft survival after transplantation remains elusive. Further, the limited pool of quality donors cannot meet the needs of the increasing number of patients on the waiting list. Strategies to expand the donor pool include liberalization of donor selection criteria, using organs from donation after cardiac death, and utilization of *ex vivo* lung perfusion. These strategies show promise in delivering more suitable organs for transplantation. Additionally, understanding the inter-dependent relationship of primary allograft dysfunction, rejection and ischemia-reperfusion injury during recovery and implantation will be key to preventing lung transplant failures.

CONSENT FOR PUBLICATION

Not applicable.

CONFLICT OF INTEREST

The authors declare no conflict of interest, financial or otherwise.

ACKNOWLEDGEMENTS

Declared none.

REFERENCES

[1]   de Perrot M, Liu M, Waddell TK, Keshavjee S. Ischemia-reperfusion-induced lung injury. Am J Respir Crit Care Med 2003; 167(4): 490-511.
[http://dx.doi.org/10.1164/rccm.200207-670SO] [PMID: 12588712]

[2]   Diamond JM, Lee JC, Kawut SM, *et al.* Clinical risk factors for primary graft dysfunction after lung transplantation. Am J Respir Crit Care Med 2013; 187(5): 527-34.
[http://dx.doi.org/10.1164/rccm.201210-1865OC] [PMID: 23306540]

[3]   de Perrot M, Bonser RS, Dark J, *et al.* Report of the ISHLT Working Group on Primary Lung Graft Dysfunction part III: donor-related risk factors and markers. J Heart Lung Transplant 2005; 24(10): 1460-7.
[http://dx.doi.org/10.1016/j.healun.2005.02.017] [PMID: 16210117]

[4]   Calhoon JK, Trinkle JK. Lung transplantation: donor selection and management. Chest Surg Clin N Am 1993; 3: 19-28.

[5]   Novick RJ, Bennett LE, Meyer DM, Hosenpud JD. Influence of graft ischemic time and donor age on survival after lung transplantation. J Heart Lung Transplant 1999; 18(5): 425-31.
[http://dx.doi.org/10.1016/S1053-2498(98)00057-6] [PMID: 10363686]

[6]   Baldwin MR, Peterson ER, Easthausen I, *et al.* Donor age and early graft failure after lung transplantation: a cohort study. Am J Transplant 2013; 13(10): 2685-95.
[http://dx.doi.org/10.1111/ajt.12428] [PMID: 24034167]

[7]   Fischer S, Gohrbandt B, Struckmeier P, *et al.* Lung transplantation with lungs from donors fifty years of age and older. J Thorac Cardiovasc Surg 2005; 129(4): 919-25.
[http://dx.doi.org/10.1016/j.jtcvs.2004.07.053] [PMID: 15821664]

[8]   Dahlman S, Jeppsson A, Scherstén H, Nilsson F. Expanding the donor pool: lung transplantation with donors 55 years and older. Transplant Proc 2006; 38(8): 2691-3.
[http://dx.doi.org/10.1016/j.transproceed.2006.07.037] [PMID: 17098041]

[9]   Bittle GJ, Sanchez PG, Kon ZN, *et al.* The use of lung donors older than 55 years: a review of the United Network of Organ Sharing database. J Heart Lung Transplant 2013; 32(8): 760-8.
[http://dx.doi.org/10.1016/j.healun.2013.04.012] [PMID: 23664760]

[10]   Holley CT, Kelly RF, Shumway SJ, *et al.* Clinical implications of donor age: A single-institution analysis spanning 3 decades. J Thorac Cardiovasc Surg 2017; 154(6): 2126-2133.e2.
[PMID: 28712587]

[11]   Katsnelson J, Whitson BA, Tumin D, *et al.* Lung transplantation with lungs from older donors: an analysis of survival in elderly recipients. J Surg Res 2017; 214: 109-16.
[http://dx.doi.org/10.1016/j.jss.2017.02.059] [PMID: 28624031]

[12]   Taghavi S, Jayarajan S, Komaroff E, *et al.* Double-lung transplantation can be safely performed using donors with heavy smoking history. Ann Thorac Surg 2013; 95: 1912-7. discussion 1917-8

[13]   Oto T, Griffiths AP, Levvey B, *et al.* A donor history of smoking affects early but not late outcome in lung transplantation. Transplantation 2004; 78(4): 599-606.
[http://dx.doi.org/10.1097/01.TP.0000131975.98323.13] [PMID: 15446321]

[14]   Yu NC, Haug MT III, Khan SU, *et al.* Does the donor-recipient ABO blood group compatibility status predict subsequent lung transplantation outcomes? J Heart Lung Transplant 1999; 18(8): 764-8.
[http://dx.doi.org/10.1016/S1053-2498(99)00034-0] [PMID: 10512522]

[15]   Taghavi S, Jayarajan SN, Furuya Y, *et al.* Examining ABO compatible donors in double lung transplants during the era of lung allocation score. Ann Thorac Surg 2014; 98(4): 1167-74.
[http://dx.doi.org/10.1016/j.athoracsur.2014.05.037] [PMID: 25106683]

[16]   Orens JB, Boehler A, de Perrot M, *et al.* A review of lung transplant donor acceptability criteria. J Heart Lung Transplant 2003; 22(11): 1183-200.

[http://dx.doi.org/10.1016/S1053-2498(03)00096-2] [PMID: 14585380]

[17]   Eberlein M, Reed RM, Bolukbas S, *et al.* Lung size mismatch and survival after single and bilateral lung transplantation 2013; 96(2): 457-63.

[18]   Meyer DM, Bennett LE, Novick RJ, Hosenpud JD. Effect of donor age and ischemic time on intermediate survival and morbidity after lung transplantation. Chest 2000; 118(5): 1255-62.
[http://dx.doi.org/10.1378/chest.118.5.1255] [PMID: 11083672]

[19]   Thabut G, Mal H, Cerrina J, *et al.* Graft ischemic time and outcome of lung transplantation: a multicenter analysis. Am J Respir Crit Care Med 2005; 171(7): 786-91.
[http://dx.doi.org/10.1164/rccm.200409-1248OC] [PMID: 15665320]

[20]   Snell GI, Rabinov M, Griffiths A, *et al.* Pulmonary allograft ischemic time: an important predictor of survival after lung transplantation. J Heart Lung Transplant 1996; 15(2): 160-8.
[PMID: 8672519]

[21]   Hennessy SA, Hranjec T, Emaminia A, *et al.* Geographic distance between donor and recipient does not influence outcomes after lung transplantation. Ann Thorac Surg 2011; 92(5): 1847-53.
[http://dx.doi.org/10.1016/j.athoracsur.2011.06.086] [PMID: 22051280]

[22]   Grimm JC, Valero V III, Kilic A, *et al.* Association between prolonged graft ischemia and primary graft failure or survival following lung transplantation. JAMA Surg 2015; 150(6): 547-53.
[http://dx.doi.org/10.1001/jamasurg.2015.12] [PMID: 25874575]

[23]   Bolton JS, Padia SA, Borja MC, *et al.* The predictive value and inter-observer variability of donor chest radiograph interpretation in lung transplantation. Eur J Cardiothorac Surg 2003; 23(4): 484-7.
[http://dx.doi.org/10.1016/S1010-7940(03)00016-2] [PMID: 12694764]

[24]   Weill D, Dey GC, Young KR, *et al.* A positive donor gram stain does not predict the development of pneumonia, oxygenation, or duration of mechanical ventilation following lung transplantation. J Heart Lung Transplant 2001; 20(2): 255. [abstract].
[http://dx.doi.org/10.1016/S1053-2498(00)00583-0] [PMID: 11250510]

[25]   Ruiz I, Gavaldà J, Monforte V, *et al.* Donor-to-host transmission of bacterial and fungal infections in lung transplantation. Am J Transplant 2006; 6(1): 178-82.
[http://dx.doi.org/10.1111/j.1600-6143.2005.01145.x] [PMID: 16433772]

CHAPTER 9

Liver Procurement: The Donor Hepatectomy

Marcos E. Pozo, Russell Wesson, Benjamin Philosophe, Andrew Cameron[*] and **Jacqueline Garonzik-Wang**

Johns Hopkins University School of Medicine, Baltimore, MD, USA

Abstract: Liver procurement is a complex surgical procedure requiring a detailed knowledge of technique, anatomy as well as anatomical variants. A thorough assessment of both the recipient and donor is necessary to optimize graft procurement, prevent complications and the possible loss of a life-saving organ. Standard liver procurement involves warm dissection of the pertinent structures followed by a rapid cold perfusion phase and subsequent evisceration. The surgical technique, as well as common pitfalls and special scenarios are discussed in this chapter with the aim of providing the reader with a comprehensive understanding of liver procurement.

Keywords: Cold Dissection, Donor Liver Procurement, Hepatic Artery Variant Anatomy, Preservation Techniques, Warm Dissection.

INTRODUCTION

Safe and efficient liver procurement is a vital component to successful liver transplantation. Given the current organ shortage, it is critical that the procuring surgeon has the expertise to safely procure a variety of liver allografts. These include livers from non-heart beating donors, expanded criteria donors and, in some instances, even splitting the liver allograft providing life-saving organs to two recipients. The purpose of this chapter is to describe the surgical steps involved in standard deceased donor liver procurement and to provide guidelines for various clinical scenarios that may arise during the procedure.

General Considerations

A successful outcome for the transplant recipient begins with the organ procurement. While the procuring surgeon is often not involved in the recipient surgical procedure, the recipient team is reliant on the judgement and technical ability of the procuring surgeon. Therefore, it is vital that the procuring surgeon take full responsibility for the assessment and safe procurement of the liver

[*] **Corresponding author Andrew Cameron:** Johns Hopkins University School of Medicine, Baltimore, MD, USA; Tel: 410502-5198; Fax: 410510-1514; Email: acamero5@jhmi.edu

Robert S.D. Higgins & Juan A. Sanchez (Eds.)

allograft. Open and frequent communication with the recipient team is paramount to ensuring a smooth and safe transplant. The procuring surgeon should also communicate preoperatively with the recipient team regarding any possible size (*i.e.* small recipient) or vascular (*i.e.* need for a conduit) concerns prior to proceeding and should follow a stepwise and systematic process to avoid any complications or allograft injuries during the procurement operation.

The donor surgeon is also responsible for a thorough pre-procurement and intra-operative evaluation of donor quality. While available information may be limited prior to arrival at the donor hospital, communication with the organ procurement organization (OPO) remains a key strategy for the well-versed transplant surgeon. Usually, a determination of the adequacy of graft has been made beforehand by the accepting transplant center. However, assessment of continued function of liver graft should be performed by the procurement team. This includes an evaluation of donor hemodynamics, oxygenation status, vasopressor requirements and type of vascular access. If there is any imaging available, it should be reviewed as it may provide information describing the presence of possible aberrant liver arterial anatomy [1].

Technique for Liver Procurement

Before Incision

The donor should be positioned supine with both arms tucked, prepped and draped to expose from the cricoid cartilage to below the symphysis pubis. This allows for maximum exposure of both thoracic and abdominal cavities. Prior to incision, the procuring surgeon should communicate with OR staff at the donor institution to ensure that all necessary equipment and instruments are available. We usually include two electrocautery and four suction devices (two Yankauer suction tips and two Poole type suction tips). We use a standard sternal retractor for the chest and a Balfour retractor for the abdominal cavity. We also converse with the local OPO ahead of time to confirm the presence of a local pathologist, should a biopsy be required.

Warm Dissection

The procedure starts with an incision extending from the xiphoid process to pubis to open the abdominal cavity (Fig. **9.1**). The round ligament is initially encountered and is divided between heavy 2-0 silk ligatures. The Balfour retractor maximizes exposure. A cruciate extension of the incision at the level of the umbilicus should be kept in mind in the case of a Balfour retractor being unavailable. In this case, the abdominal wall flaps can be secured laterally with penetrating towel clips. The falciform ligament is divided back to the inferior vena cava-hepatic vein confluence. Abdominal cavity evaluation should then be performed to evaluate for any absolute or relative contraindications to procurement. These include: malignancy, active peritonitis or hollow viscus perforation, cirrhosis or other liver disease. The liver should be assessed carefully for quality and if there is any concern, the procuring surgeon should have a low threshold to proceed with biopsy and rapid histologic assessment. Once the quality of the liver is assessed and deemed acceptable, the surgeon can proceed with the remainder of the procurement. If we are waiting on biopsy results, we proceed with the warm dissection, but do not transition to the cold dissection until we confirm that we have indeed accepted the liver for our intended recipient.

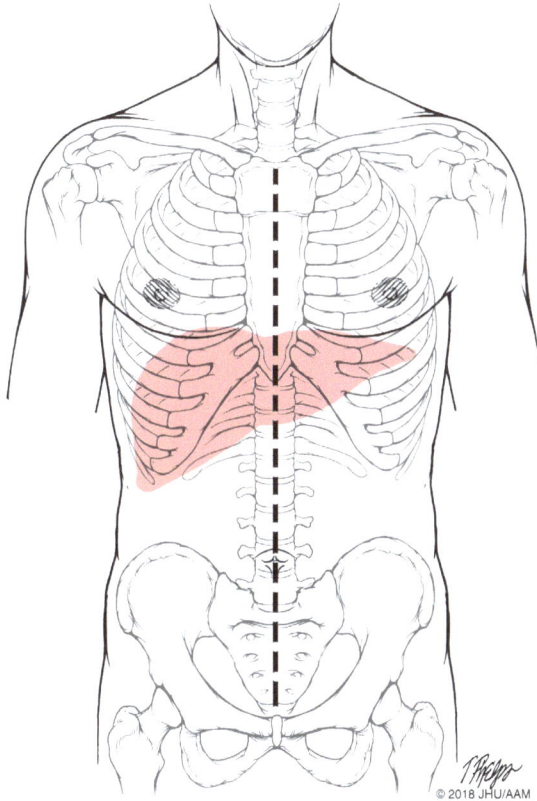

Fig. (9.1). The procedure starts with an incision extending from the xiphoid process to pubis to open the abdominal cavity. Medical Illustrations© 2018 Tim Phelps, MS, FAMI, Johns Hopkins University.

Next, we expose the aorta and inferior mesenteric vein (IMV) in anticipation of vessel cannulation. The right colon is mobilized extensively (Catell-Braash maneuver), including kocherization of the duodenum (Fig. **9.2**). During this process care should be taken to avoid injuring the right ureter. We often identify it and encircle it with a vessel loop, to protect against injury during the process of aortic exposure. This visceral mobilization is continued to the ligament of Treitz. After completion of this maneuver, the surgeon should be able to identify the aorta and inferior vena cava (IVC), the left renal vein traversing to the IVC across the Aorta and the IMV in the mesentery just to the left of the ligament of Treitz (Fig. **9.3**). At this point, we encircle the aorta with two umbilical tapes to prepare for cannulation later. The aorta should be encircled just above the iliac bifurcation and the surgeon should clear enough distance (usually ~2 cm) to safely cannulate the aorta. Care should be taken to avoid injuring the IVC or any lumbar arteries as well as any low-lying renal arteries. A small percentage of patients will have renal arteries originating from the distal aorta or iliac arteries and the procuring surgeon must be vigilant for this variant. Next, we identify and encircle the inferior mesenteric vein with two silk ties in preparation for future cannulation. Some surgeons cannulate the IMV at this point and initiate pre-cool.

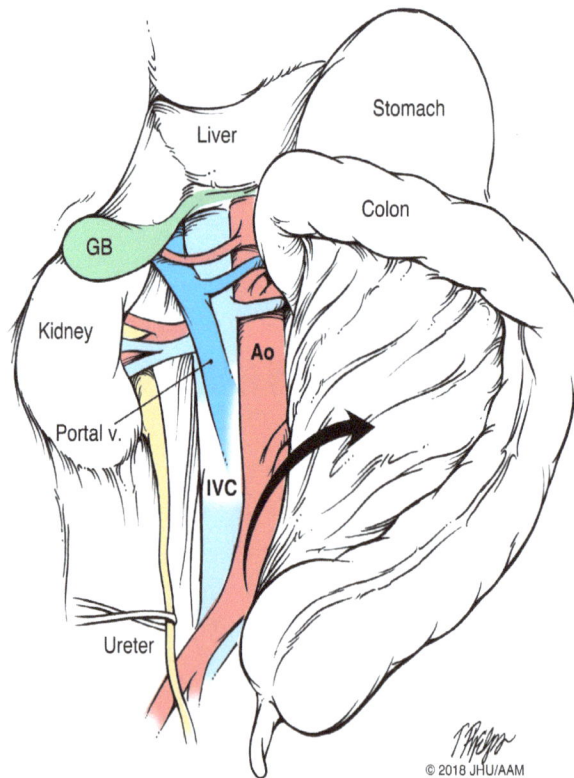

Fig. (9.2). The right colon is mobilized extensively (Catell-Braash maneuver), including kocherization of the duodenum. Medical Illustrations© 2018 Tim Phelps, MS, FAMI, Johns Hopkins University.

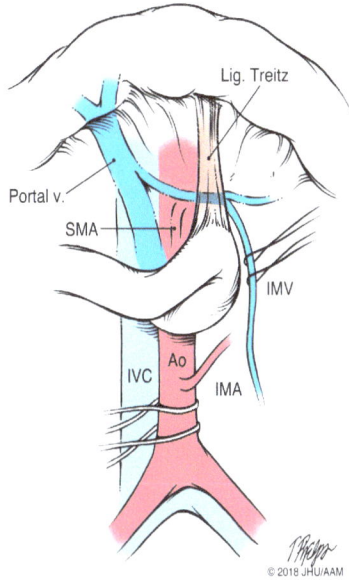

Fig. (9.3). Identification of the aorta and inferior vena cava (IVC), the left renal vein traversing to the IVC across the Aorta and the IMV in the mesentery just to the left of the ligament of Treitz. Medical Illustrations© 2018 Tim Phelps, MS, FAMI, Johns Hopkins University.

Next, the surgeons should expose and mobilize the liver and the portal structures. First the left lateral segment should be mobilized by exposing and cauterizing the left triangular ligament. This will allow for elevation of the left lateral segment. Next the gastrohepatic ligament is examined carefully for a possible replaced or accessory left hepatic artery arising from the left gastric artery (Fig. **9.4**). If confirmed, dissection should proceed 5 mm above and below it (parallel to the replaced artery) to preserve the variant vessel.

Next, we turn our attention the porta hepatis. Dissection of the porta hepatis begins with careful palpation determining if there is either a replaced right hepatic artery or in some instances an entirely replaced arterial system. Any pulsation on the lateral or posterior border of the common bile duct (CBD) should raise the alert for a possible replaced right hepatic artery (Fig. **9.4**). After this maneuver, the next step is to identify and encircle the common bile duct (CBD). Care should be taken to avoid any arterial aberrant anatomy coursing posterior to the CBD. Additionally, all portal dissection should proceed far from the hepatic hilum and close to the donor duodenum, in order to preserve length on all of the pertinent structures. We tie the CBD with a silk ligature distally, close to the duodenum and then incise the CBD just proximal to the silk tie. Next, the fundus of the gallbladder is opened and an Asepto irrigation bulb syringe is utilized to flush the gallbladder and CBD with saline, until the effluent has cleared. If there is a stone in the gallbladder blocking flow or the donor has had a previous cholecystectomy, we will use a pediatric feeding tube attached to a 60 cc syringe and flush the CBD in a retrograde fashion.

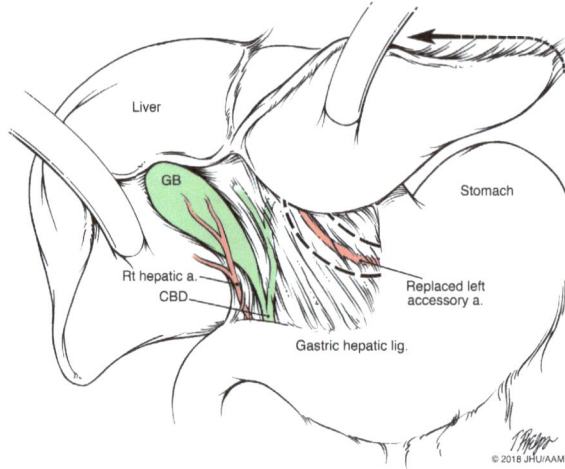

Fig. (9.4). Any pulsation on the lateral or posterior border of the common bile duct (CBD) should raise the alert for a possible replaced right hepatic artery. Medical Illustrations© 2018 Tim Phelps, MS, FAMI, Johns Hopkins University.

Next, we identify the common hepatic artery by elevating the common hepatic artery lymph node. If there is normal arterial anatomy, the artery is almost always located immediately below the lymph node. We elect to perform minimal dissection of the hepatic artery in the warm dissection, in order to not injure it and risk inadequate hepatic arterial flush. We expose enough in the warm so that we are confident we can safely identify and trace out the artery in the cold portion of the dissection. Finally, we expose the supraceliac aorta in anticipation of cannulation, cold perfusion and cross-clamp. The left lateral segment of the liver is retracted to the patient's right and the esophagus and stomach are pulled toward the patient's left side. This maneuver will expose the diaphragmatic crura (Fig. **9.5**). The crura are incised with electrocautery to the level of the supraceliac aorta. The surgeon can either encircle the aorta with an umbilical tape to aid in cross-clamp or expose enough aorta so that a vascular clamp be placed around the aorta in its entirety. If the surgeon elects not to encircle the aorta, a clamp can be placed around the aorta until the tips of the clamp are felt pressing against the vertebral body (the posterior most extent of the aorta) and closed at the time of cross-clamp. The thoracic cavity exposure and exploration will either be performed by the thoracic or cardiac team or by the abdominal surgeon if no thoracic organs are being procured. Thoracic exposure and dissection are described elsewhere in this book.

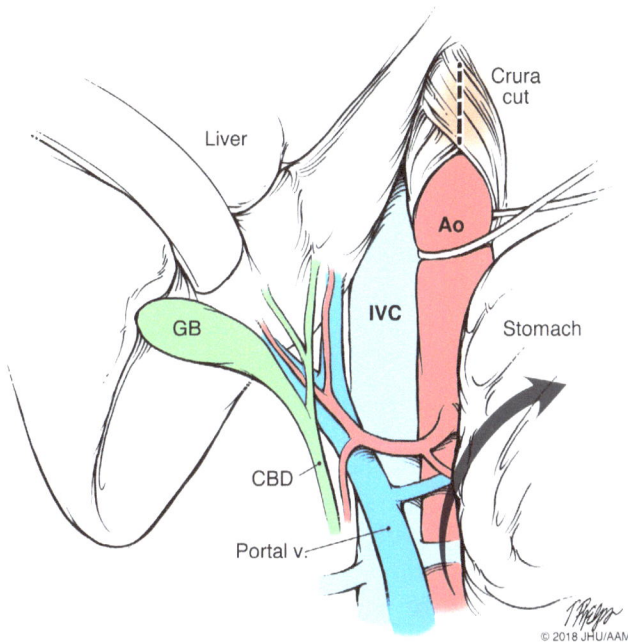

Fig. (9.5). The diaphragmatic crura is exposed after the left lateral segment of the liver is retracted to the patient's right and the esophagus and stomach are pulled toward the patients left side. Medical Illustrations© 2018 Tim Phelps, MS, FAMI, Johns Hopkins University.

This completes the exposure portion of the warm dissection and steps are taken to transition to the cold dissection. A single dose of 30,000 units of heparin is administered by the anesthesia team and allowed to circulate for approximately 3 minutes. During this time, the IMV cannula (for portal flush) can be inserted. The distal IMV is ligated with a silk tie. Just proximal to the tie, a small venotomy is made in the IMV and the cannula is inserted. This is secured with a silk tie on the superior portion of the IMV. We use a 10 Fr portal cannula; however, some centers opt to use an IV cannula or smaller tubing. After the heparin has circulated for three minutes, we proceed with aortic cannulation. We take the inferior previously placed umbilical tape and ligate the aorta just above the bifurcation. The superior umbilical tape is pulled up in the air by the assistant and the surgeon compresses the aorta at the same level with their fingers. An aortotomy is made just above the tied umbilical tape and the aortic cannula is inserted. This is secured with the superior umbilical tape. We use a 24Fr aortic cannula, however if the donor is small, we often ask our OPO staff to have a 20Fr or 18Fr available. This completes the warm dissection.

Organ Cold Perfusion

Before allowing preservation solutions to bathe the liver, appropriate communication with OPO coordinator and anesthesia team is held to ensure all members of the team are aware cross-clamp and cold perfusion are imminent. All hollow viscus should be returned to abdominal cavity to prevent torsion, spasm or occlusion of cannulas. Expeditiously, the surgeon places the clamp on the supraceliac aorta, transects the vena cava at the junction of the right atrium and IVC to allow venting or exsanguination while cannulas are opened widely (Fig. **9.6**). We use University of Wisconsin (UW) Solution for preservation and often instill 3L via the aortic cannula and 2L *via* the portal cannula. Some centers utilize HTK solution, in which case the standard perfusate volume is 5L in the aortic cannula and 3L in the portal cannula [2, 3]. Higher volumes are usually recommended for non-heart beating donors, as it often takes longer to gain access to and cross-clamp the aorta and the IMV may not be cannulated. Next, ice is placed over the liver and in the paracolic gutters over the kidneys. The lesser sac should be packed with ice as well if pancreas is being procured. During cold perfusion, there is often downtime to remove mesenteric lymph nodes, which are later utilized for retrospective crossmatch.

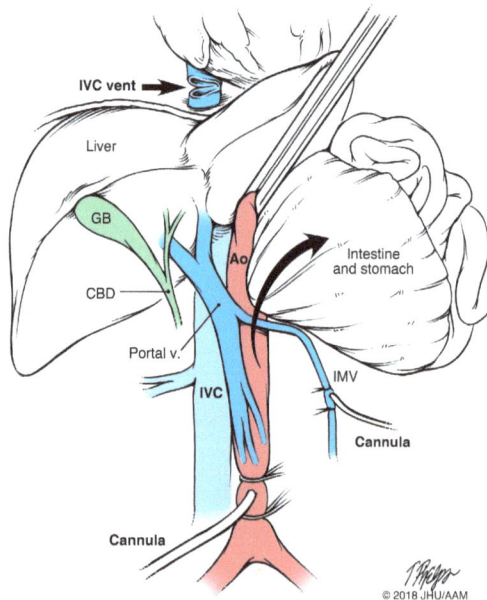

Fig. (9.6). The surgeon places the clamp on the supraceliac aorta, transects the vena cava at the junction of the right atrium and IVC to allow venting or exsanguination while cannulas are opened widely. Medical Illustrations© 2018 Tim Phelps, MS, FAMI, Johns Hopkins University.

Cold Dissection

After cold perfusion, we turn our attention to the liver procurement. The cold dissection begins, first by cutting the right and left hemi-diaphragms, from the anterior reflection to the posterior abdominal wall. This proceeds at least a few centimeters lateral to the suprahepatic cava to prevent caval or hepatic injury. After this maneuver, the liver will gently fall into the chest. We place ice in the chest prior to this, so the liver has a cold surface to lay on. We also lower the liver into the chest slowly while simultaneously examining the undersurface of the liver. There are usually peritoneal attachments between the inferior surface of the liver and the retroperitoneum. These need to be sharply divided so the liver capsule is not ripped as the liver falls into the chest. Next, we place a Poole tip suction behind the porta hepatis from right to left to elevate the portal structures (Fig. **9.7**). Ligation of the superficially located right gastric artery allows for exposure of the gastroduodenal artery (GDA) which is encountered first at the superior edge of duodenum. The GDA is ligated distally, near the pancreas border to maintain length in case it is needed for vascular reconstruction. Next, we encounter the portal vein, which is often posterior to the GDA (Fig. **9.8**). If the pancreas is not being procured (pancreas procurement is discussed elsewhere in this text), we bluntly create a tunnel under the head of the pancreas and bivalve the pancreas. This exposes the retro-pancreatic portal vein and the confluence of the splenic and superior mesenteric vein. We transect the splenic and superior mesenteric vein to ensure adequate length of the portal vein (Fig. **9.9**).

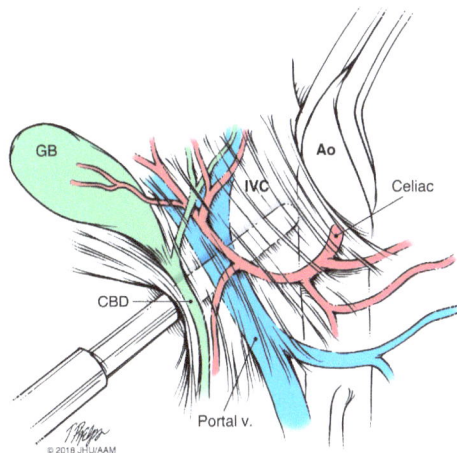

Fig. (9.7). A Poole tip suction is placed behind the porta hepatis from right to left to elevate the portal structures. Medical Illustrations© 2018 Tim Phelps, MS, FAMI, Johns Hopkins University.

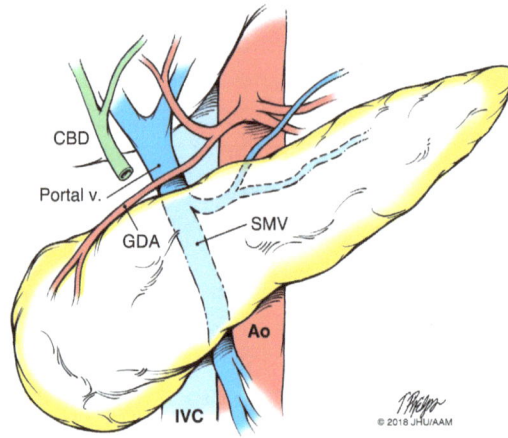

Fig. (9.8). The portal vein is often posterior to the GDA. Medical Illustrations© 2018 Tim Phelps, MS, FAMI, Johns Hopkins University.

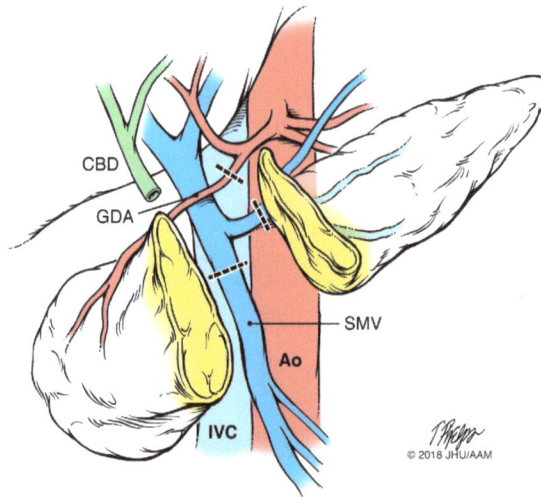

Fig. (9.9). The splenic and superior mesenteric veins are transected to ensure adequate length of the portal vein. Medical Illustrations© 2018 Tim Phelps, MS, FAMI, Johns Hopkins University.

Next, we proceed with the arterial dissection. We expose the hepatic artery and trace it back to the celiac axis where the left gastric and splenic artery come off. If there is a replaced left hepatic artery, the safest way to preserve this is to sharply divide all of the mesentery from the superior portion of the lesser curve of the stomach, taking care to stay exceedingly close to the stomach. The left gastric artery travels in this tissue and if one stays close to the stomach injury is avoided.

If there is a replaced right hepatic artery, this should be preserved during the portal dissection. Next, the splenic artery is traced toward the pancreas and is transected within the pancreas. The splenic artery can then be gently held straight up in the air and serves as the medial border of further dissection. The celiac is then traced to the level of the aorta and removed with a Carrell patch of aorta (Fig. **9.10**). If there is a replaced right hepatic artery, the Carrell patch should include the superior mesenteric artery (SMA) from which the replaced right originates.

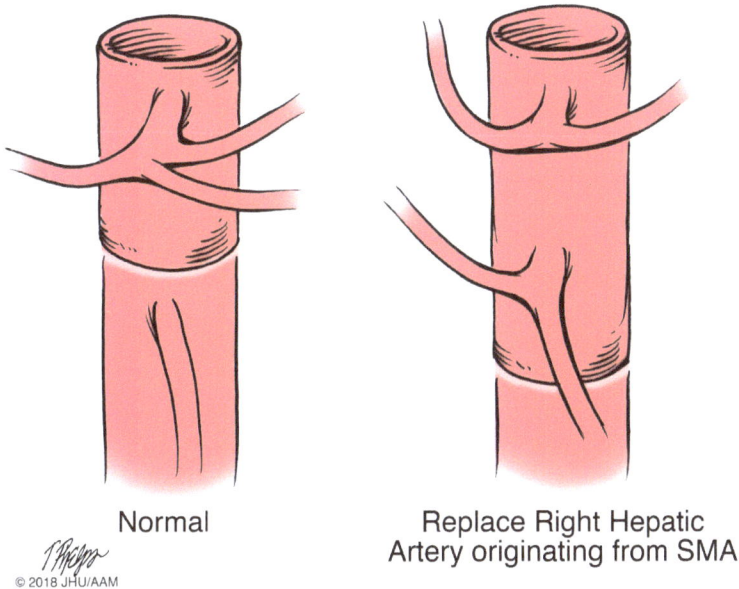

Normal

Replace Right Hepatic
Artery originating from SMA

© 2018 JHU/AAM

Fig. (9.10). The celiac is then traced to the level of the aorta and removed with a Carrell patch of aorta. Medical Illustrations© 2018 Tim Phelps, MS, FAMI, Johns Hopkins University.

Finally, the infrahepatic cava must be transected. Care is taken to identify the left and right renal veins and transect the IVC leaving at least a 3-5 mm margin above the right renal vein. After caval transection, the liver is separated from the remaining retroperitoneal attachments. The procuring surgeon should displace the right kidney inferiorly with one hand and transect these attachments by cutting through the middle of the right adrenal gland. This prevents injury to both the liver and the right kidney. The liver is then mobilized circumferentially, and any remaining attachments are transected. During this process, the surgeon should place one finger in the suprahepatic cava to precisely know its position and protect from injury while the other hand covers and protect the portal structures. The liver is then passed off to the backtable and placed in cold preservation solution. It is examined for any anatomical abnormalities or injuries and then packaged according to OPO and preservation protocols. The abdominal procurement team has the final task of harvesting any additional lymph nodes and/or the spleen and the iliac vessels for possible vascular reconstruction [4].

Special Scenarios

Unexpected Intraabdominal Findings

Certain scenarios may be encountered by the procurement team that require modification of the previously described standard liver procurement technique. In cases of peritonitis diagnosed upon entry to abdominal cavity, intra-operative cultures and emergent Gram stain should be performed. Most centers advocate for broad spectrum antibiotic coverage to recipient until culture data is finalized. Incidentally found malignancies are not uncommon and any observed mass should be sent for pathology and the recipient team should be notified immediately.

Alternative Cannulation and Cross-Clamp Sites

In circumstances where the infrarenal aorta is very diseased, alternative cannulation sites include the iliac arteries or the ascending or descending thoracic aorta. Additionally, if the donor has had a previous sternotomy, the donor surgeon should perform all of the warm dissection and cannulation prior to opening the chest. In this instance, the heart is often stuck to the sternum and injured during sternotomy. Alternative sites for venous venting include the IVC just above the iliac bifurcation. A small venotomy should be made and a pool sucker can be placed in the cava. Finally, if supraceliac cross clamp of the aorta is not feasible, one can access the descending thoracic aorta in the chest by ligating the inferior pulmonary ligament on the left and bluntly transecting the pleura anterior to the aorta. This can be found by palpating for the first round, pulsating structure anterior to the vertebral body. We often cross-clamp in the chest if the donor has a replaced left hepatic artery so tension is not placed on this vessel.

Donation after Cardiac Death (DCD)

Full description of DCD procurement is outside of the scope of this chapter. However, several important considerations are outlined below. First, the procuring and recipient surgeon should discuss ahead of time the important parameters they will use in determining if the donor progressed in satisfactory proximity to withdraw of life support. Some centers only consider time; however, many transplant surgeons will only include agonal time in their consideration (*i.e.* time spent when the donor is significantly hypotensive or hypoxic). The majority of transplant centers will accept a DCD with warm ischemia time that is less than 30-45 minutes from withdrawal of support to cold perfusion [5, 6]. If the patient progresses, each OPO has a pre-determined asystole time that must pass to confirm the absence of auto-resuscitation, prior to incision. It is pertinent that the procuring surgeon not be involved in any determination of time of death or in the care of the donor prior to the incision. This should be determined by a practitioner unrelated to the transplant team and avoids conflict of interest. Heparin should be given around the time of withdrawal, in case the patient progresses and the OPO often manages this based on their protocols and procedures. Once the patient has been pronounced by the declaring practitioner, procurement proceeds very rapidly. A long midline incision is made with the scalpel, and often heavy Mayo scissors are used to rapidly open the peritoneal cavity. The colon is sharply mobilized and the aorta is identified and cannulated. Cold perfusion is immediately started. We subsequently make a venotomy in the IVC and place a Poole sucker within it to vent venous blood. We then elect to expose and cannulate the IMV for portal perfusion, however some surgeons only do a large volume aortic flush and perform a portal flush on the backtable. The chest is then opened and the aorta is cross-clamped. All of this should occur within 5-10 minutes. Next the gallbladder should be incised and the CBD transected. The gallbladder and CBD should be flushed with saline in the same fashion as mentioned above. The remainder of the procurement proceeds as described above. The organ should be thoroughly examined on the backtable to rule out any iatrogenic injury.

CONCLUSION

The responsibility of the procuring team in liver transplantation cannot be understated. The optimal donor hepatectomy procedure is safe and efficient, and it is fundamentally based on excellent communication between all team members to ensure no unwarranted loss of scarce resources given our current organ shortage. Furthermore, the transplant surgeon must be well-versed in variant anatomy, and be able to adapt to a variety of liver allografts including non-heart beating donors and expanded criteria donors.

CONSENT FOR PUBLICATION

Not applicable.

CONFLICT OF INTEREST

The author declares no conflict of interest, financial or otherwise.

ACKNOWLEDGEMENTS

Declared none.

REFERENCES

[1]   Cameron AM, Yersiz H, Busuttil RW. Liver donation: surgical techniques. Transplant Rev 2005; 19(2): 108-14.
[http://dx.doi.org/10.1016/j.trre.2005.06.001]

[2]   García-Gil FA, Serrano MT, Fuentes-Broto L, *et al.* Celsior versus University of Wisconsin preserving solutions for liver transplantation: postreperfusion syndrome and outcome of a 5-year prospective randomized controlled study. World J Surg 2011; 35(7): 1598-607.
[http://dx.doi.org/10.1007/s00268-011-1078-7] [PMID: 21487851]

[3]   Cavallari A, Cillo U, Nardo B, *et al.* A multicenter pilot prospective study comparing Celsior and University of Wisconsin preserving solutions for use in liver transplantation. Liver Transpl 2003; 9(8): 814-21.
[http://dx.doi.org/10.1053/jlts.2003.50161] [PMID: 12884193]

[4]   Eghtesad B, Kadry Z, Fung J. Technical considerations in liver transplantation: what a hepatologist needs to know (and every surgeon should practice). Liver Transpl 2005 Aug; 11(8): 861-71.

[5]   Reich DJ, Mulligan DC, Abt PL, *et al.* ASTS recommended practice guidelines for controlled donation after cardiac death organ procurement and transplantation. Am J Transplant 2009; 9(9): 2004-11.
[http://dx.doi.org/10.1111/j.1600-6143.2009.02739.x] [PMID: 19624569]

[6]   Mandell M. Executive summary from the intraoperative advisory council on donation after cardiac death of the united network for organ sharing: practice guidelines. Liver Transplantation 2003 Oct; 9(10): 1120-3.

CHAPTER 10

Organ Specific Considerations: Pancreas and Kidney

Iyore James, Ashraf El-Hinnawi and **Amer Rajab**[*]

The Ohio State University, Columbus, OH, USA

Abstract: Pancreas transplantation is experiencing a resurgence in interest as one of the last frontiers in multiorgan transplantation. Most commonly performed in combination with kidney transplantation, this chapter reviews key aspects of donor assessment as well as preservation and anatomic recovery to enhance success of these procedures. Pancreas transplantation in Donation after cardiac death is also reviewed as an evolving potential source of organs in this field.

Keywords: Donation after Cardiac Death (DCD), Donation of Pancreas, Kidney Transplant, Pancreas Transplant.

INTRODUCTION

Diabetes is a leading cause of end stage kidney disease (ESKD) requiring renal replacement therapy. End-stage kidney disease is a significant cause of morbidity and mortality. Death from kidney disease is the ninth leading cause of death in the United States [1]. Of the 96,681 patients waiting for a kidney transplant, less than 20% of candidates on the kidney transplant list receive a kidney due to organ shortage [2]. Therefore, it is very important to maximize utilization of kidneys by encouraging living donation and improve utilization of deceased donor kidneys by proper organ selection, procurement and preservation.

After a decade of steady decline in pancreas transplantation, the last three years have seen a stable number of pancreas transplants being performed annually in the United States. The total number of deceased donors in the United States over the last 5 years was 44,058 with a pancreas procurement rate of 15.3%. Of those pancreata procured, only 75% was used for transplant [3]. Pancreas transplantation is most commonly performed in combination with kidney transplantation. Diabetic patients who will require dialysis and who experience hypoglycemic unawareness are ideal candidates for simultaneous pancreas kidney

[*] **Corresponding author Amer Rajab:** The Ohio State University, Columbus, OH, USA Tel: 614-293-6322; Fax: 614-293-4541; Email: amer.rajab@osumc.edu

Robert S.D. Higgins & Juan A. Sanchez (Eds.)

transplant (SPKT). Pancreas transplantation may also be performed alone or as a procedure after kidney transplant. Appropriate donor selection, proper recovery and preservation of the pancreas are of utmost importance in achieving excellent outcomes.

Donor Selection [Pancreas]

Donation after brain death (DBD) constitutes 95% of pancreas donors. Highly selected donation after cardiac death (DCD) and living donation collectively constitute less than 5% of pancreas donors.

The ideal deceased pancreas donor is between 18 and 34 years of age with a normal BMI (less than $35kg/m^2$), no medical comorbidities and death from a traumatic injury. The proportion of "non-ideal" pancreas donors is increasing corresponding to a higher incidence of discarded pancreatic allografts due to donor BMI greater than 35 kg/m^2 [2].

Pancreas allografts may also be obtained from deceased pediatric donors. In a study from the Ohio State University Transplant Comprehensive Center, simultaneous kidney pancreas transplant (SPKT) recipients receiving allografts from pediatric donors had comparable short and long-term outcomes as SPKT recipients who received allografts from ideal age donors. Furthermore, there was no increased incidence of technical failure with pediatric allografts [4].

Absolute contraindications for using pancreas from a deceased donor are: hemoglobin A-1 C greater than 6 which indicates a diabetic donor; BMI greater than 40 kg/m_2; age greater than 60 years and intra-operative evaluation demonstrating evidence of trauma, fibrosis, inflammation or fatty infiltration of the pancreas. Donor hyperglycemia or hyperamylasemia are not contraindications to utilizing a pancreatic allograft for transplant.

Donor Selection [Kidney]

Approximately 70% of kidney transplants performed in the United States are from deceased donors [5]. The proportion of donation after cardiac death (DCD) kidneys increased from 7.3% in 2005 to 17.7% in 2015 [6]. A policy enabling the use of extended criteria donor (ECD) kidneys (donor age ≥60 years or 50 to 59 years with at least two of the following: history of hypertension, serum creatinine level >1.5 mg/dL, or cerebrovascular cause of death) was implemented in November 2000 in an attempt to increase the donor pool and improve patient survival from dialysis-dependent ESKD. An ECD kidney has a 70% greater likelihood of graft loss when compared to a SCD kidney, however receiving an ECD kidney carries significant survival benefit compared to remaining on dialysis. In 2012, the Organ Procurement and Transplantation Network (OPTN) introduced the Kidney Donor Profile Index (KDPI), which compiles 10 donor factors (instead of four in the ECD definition) that are independently associated with all-cause allograft survival associated with the use of that organ. A donor KDPI >85% is thought to be equivalent to an ECD kidney. The KDPI was the basis of the new allocation policy introduced toward the end of 2014 to increase the utilization of marginal kidneys and decrease the discard rates that would be expected when using the older ECD classification [7].

Procurement

Prior to abdominal organ recovery, it is adamant that the donor surgeon reviews the donor chart to confirm identity of the donor and other relevant facts such the correct ABO type, serologies, presence of transmissible diseases, lab values to ensure functioning organs and, donor comorbidities that may impact graft function. In some high-risk donors, kidney graft biopsy may be required prior to transplantation.

The kidney and pancreas are typically procured as part of a multi-organ procurement procedure but can be recovered alone. Before starting the multi-organ procurement, it is mandatory that the different surgical teams discuss the techniques and sequences they want to adopt.

The principle of organ procurement is the core cooling of the organs to be removed and flushing the organs with preservative solution to mitigate cellular damage. Various preservation solutions and protocols exist with widespread variability among transplant centers.

The surgical procedure for DBD donors is initiated by a midline laparotomy including a sternotomy with optional transverse laparotomy at the level of the umbilicus to gain access to the abdominal and thoracic organs, a sternotomy can be spared in certain circumstances, such as previous cardiothoracic surgeries, if only abdominal organs are to be procured (Fig. **10.1**). Organs are inspected for anatomy, viability, and to exclude obvious malignancies. The vascular anatomy to the liver and pancreas is evaluated to assess for accessory or replaced right or left hepatic arteries as this may impact the surgical technique. Minimal liver hilar dissection is required to identify the common and proper hepatic arteries, gastroduodenal artery (GDA), splenic (SA) artery and the common bile duct (CBD); this is necessary to minimize the risk of injury and time for removing the pancreas. The small and large intestines are mobilized to gain access to the retroperitoneum. The aorta is exposed at its bifurcation in preparation for cannulation; the inferior mesenteric vein is exposed for portal venous flush. The pancreas and spleen are dissected en-bloc, all the splenic ligaments are divided;

the lesser curvature of the stomach is divided and the body and tail of the pancreas are dissected free from the retroperitoneum. Care must be taken not to violate the pancreas or injure the splenic vessels. The aortic cross-clamp site is identified either at the supra celiac aorta in the abdomen (if thoracic organs are being procured or to avoid a sternotomy) or the descending aorta in the chest. In preparation for cross-clamp, the patient is heparinized with 30,000 to 50,000 units of heparin intravenously and allowed to circulate for 3 minutes. The aortic cannula is placed; the aorta is cross-clamped; flushing of the organs with cold preservative solution is initiated and a hole is made in the inferior vena cava (IVC) for drainage or the right atrium if a sternotomy is made. The organs to be procured should be cooled by placing ice cold slush in the abdominal cavity.

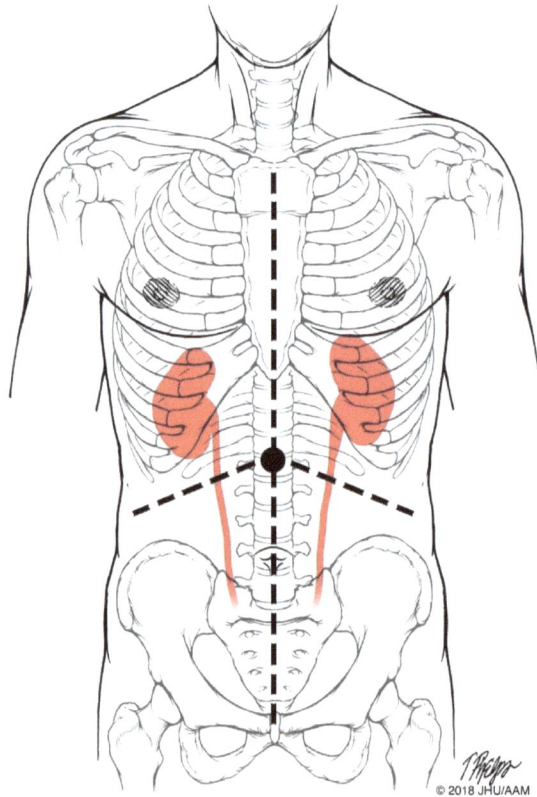

Fig. (10.1). The surgical procedure for DBD donors is initiated by a midline laparotomy including a sternotomy with optional transverse laparotomy at the level of the umbilicus to gain access to the abdominal and thoracic organs. Medical Illustrations© 2018 Tim Phelps, MS, FAMI, Johns Hopkins University.

After completion of flushing, dissection and organ removal should be done expeditiously and smoothly to minimize organ damage. The pancreas, spleen and duodenum can be removed en-bloc with the liver and separated at the back table or removed alone after the liver is procured (the decision is based on surgeon preference). The goal is to remove the organ expeditiously while avoiding organ injury.

The portal vein is divided between the pancreas and the liver with care not to shorten the portal vein on the pancreas side (Fig. **10.2**). The SA and superior mesenteric artery (SMA) are cut and divided at their origin with care taken to assess the presence of an accessory or replaced right hepatic artery originating from the SMA, which will need to be preserved. In this instance, division of the SMA will be above the branching point of the right replaced or accessory hepatic artery. In certain situations, the right replaced or accessory hepatic artery may course in the parenchyma of the head of the pancreas. If so present, in order to preserve the integrity of the pancreas, the right replaced or accessory hepatic artery must be divided just distal to the head of the pancreas toward the hilum of the liver and ligated proximally. The duodenum is then stapled proximally and distally (Fig. **10.3**).

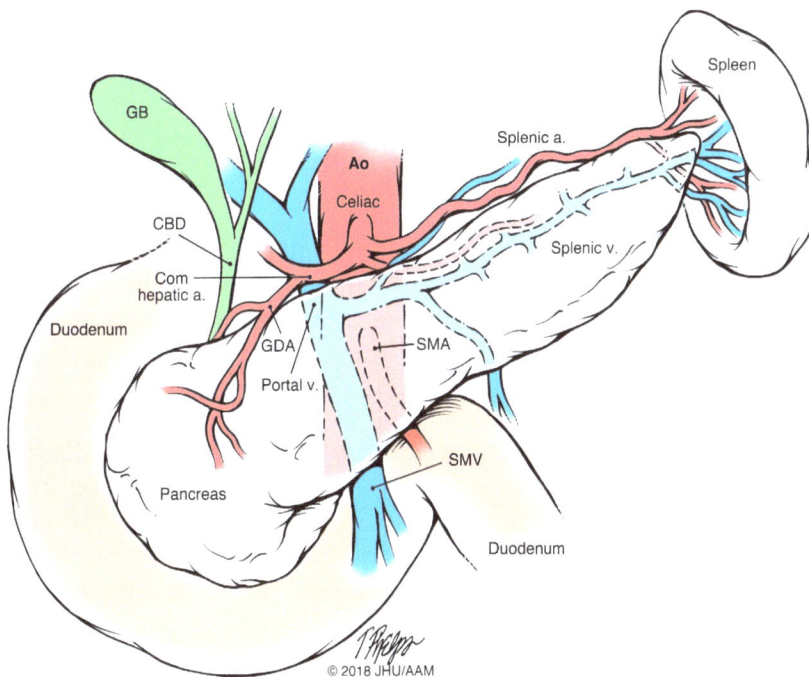

Fig. (10.2). The pancreas is removed en-bloc with the spleen and duodenum. Liver not shown. Medical Illustrations© 2018 Tim Phelps, MS, FAMI, Johns Hopkins University.

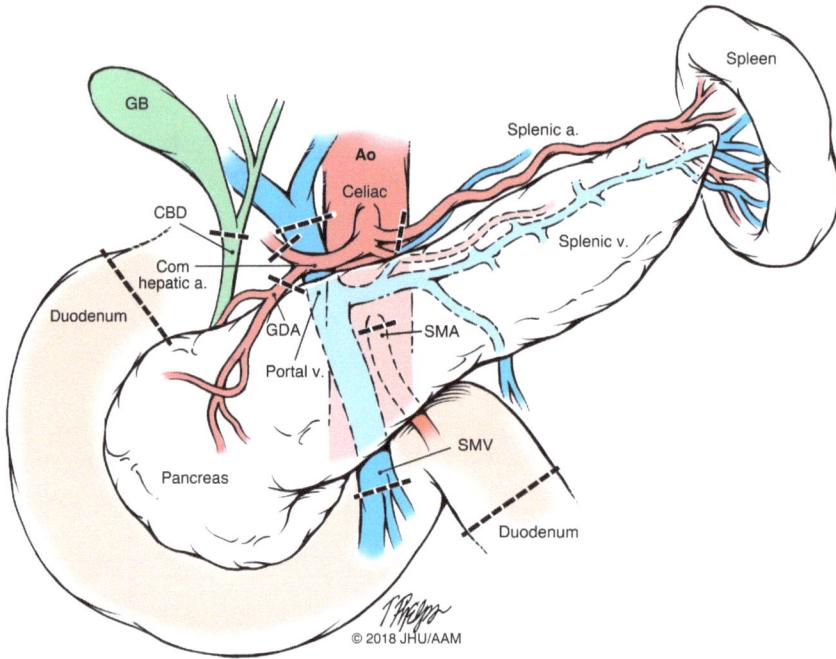

Fig. (10.3). The CBD and GDA are ligated and divided extra pancreatic. The portal vein is divided between the pancreas and the liver; take care not to shorten the portal vein on the pancreas side. The duodenum is shortened to length. Medical Illustrations© 2018 Tim Phelps, MS, FAMI, Johns Hopkins University.

The spleen will serve as a handle to minimize manipulation and injury to the pancreas during transplant and it also maintains adequate inflow and outflow of the pancreas allograft immediately after transplant. The spleen is removed at the time of transplant after the drainage of the duodenum is completed and the vasospasm of the pancreatic vessels resolve.

The kidneys are removed separately or en bloc to be separated on the back table. The ureters are divided as close to the bladder as possible. The kidneys are dissected free from Gerota's fascia. The IVC and aorta are divided at the bifurcation and retracted anteriorly and superiorly and, sharply dissected free from the spine to remove the kidneys. The left renal vein is divided at the junction with the IVC, the aorta is opened vertically on the anterior and posterior surface between the paired lumbar vessels to allow visualization of renal arteries orifices and avoid renal artery injury. The fat should be cleaned cautiously from the kidney to identify any gross abnormality; the anatomy of the kidney should be checked and reported.

The common, external and internal iliac arteries (CIA, EIA, IIA) and veins are also procured to use for vascular reconstruction. The CIA, EIA and IIA are used as a Y graft for arterial reconstruction of pancreas allograft by connecting the EIA to SMA and IIA to SA creating a single inflow vessel to the pancreas. Lymph nodes and spleen are also procured for purpose of tissue typing and cross match.

Controlled DCD procurement has the same general principles. Life support is withdrawn in a controlled environment. Organ procurement is allowed when the patient is asystolic for 5 minutes and pronounced dead by another physician that is not part of the procurement team. Time from withdrawal of care to asystole is measured, and if this warm ischemia time is accepted by the transplant center (most centers will accept up to 60 minutes for kidney or pancreas procurement) then procurement proceeds. At this point access to the infra renal aorta, cannulation, flushing, supraceliac or thoracic aortic cross clamp and venting through the IVC in the abdomen or the right atrium should be done as quickly as possible to minimize warm ischemia time. The remaining dissection is done in situ as previously described for DBD donors. Care must be exercised to identify all the necessary structures to prevent organ damage or injury.

Preservation

Preservation solutions differ in composition yet share similar objectives of reducing graft edema, intracellular acidosis, production of reactive active oxygen species, and providing energy substrates for metabolism. Histidine-tryptopha--ketoglutarate (HTK), University of Wisconsin solution (UW) and Celsius (CE) are the most common used preservative solutions. No difference was observed with these preservation solutions with respect to graft and patient survival [8].

Studies reveal that UW, HTK, and CE are equivalent with respect to patient and graft survival in renal and pancreas transplants. In addition, kidney delayed graft function appears to be comparable for UW, HTK, and CE. UW solution is favored in pancreas transplants given the concern for pancreatitis and graft thrombosis associated with HTK [8].

The organs are preserved in a preservative solution in an ice-cold environment. The pancreas can tolerate up to 24 hours of cold ischemia time. The kidneys can tolerate up to 24 hours of static cold ischemia time and up to 72 hours on Hypothermic Pulsatile machine perfusion.

Cold static storage remains the most dominant method for renal preservation having surpassed machine perfusion in the 1980s due to lack of evidence demonstrating improved outcomes and increased costs. However, the persistent organ shortage and the ever-changing donor profile have generated interest in machine perfusion. In an international randomized control trial, hypothermic machine perfusion was associated with a reduce risk of delayed graft function and improved graft survival following kidney transplantation [9, 10]. Hypothermic machine perfusion has also been shown to reduce delayed graft function and primary non function in extended criteria donor kidneys [11, 12].

CONCLUSION/FUTURE DIRECTION

Advances in preservative and perfusion technology have led to increased graft utilization, increased viability assessment and improved graft survival in kidney, liver and heart transplantation. Unfortunately, these benefits have not translated to pancreas transplantation. Further studies are needed to optimize machine perfusion for pancreatic allografts.

Islet cell transplantation remains a viable alternative to whole pancreas transplant. The Edmonton Protocol has led to multiple clinical trials whereby isolated islet cells from deceased donor pancreas allografts are infused into the recipient's portal vein [13]. Clinical studies to optimize islet cell delivery are essential to decrease need for multiple islet cell transplants and provide long-term insulin independence.

CONSENT FOR PUBLICATION

Not applicable.

CONFLICT OF INTEREST

The authors declare no conflict of interest, financial or otherwise.

ACKNOWLEDGEMENTS

Declared none.

REFERENCES

[1]   Kochanek KD, Murphy SL, Xu JQ, *et al.* Deaths: final data for 2014. http://wwwcdcgov 2016 June 30; Accessed September 5, 2017

[2]   OPTN Data https://optntransplanthrsagov/data

[3]   Kandaswamy R, Stock PG, Gustafson SK, *et al.* OPTN/SRTR 2015 Annual Data Report: Pancreas. Am J Transplant 2017; 17 (Suppl. 1): 117-73.
[http://dx.doi.org/10.1111/ajt.14125] [PMID: 28052606]

[4]   El-Hinnawi A, Elkhammas E, Pelletier R, *et al.* Pediatric Donors for Simultaneous Pancreas-Kidney Transplant (SPKT). Presented at World Transplant Congress 2014. 2014 July; California, United States. San Francisco 2014.

[5]   United Network for Organ Sharing (UNOS). https://www.unos.org/data/transplant-trends Accessed September 5, 2017

[6]   Hart A, Smith JM, Skeans MA, *et al.* OPTN/SRTR 2015 Annual data report: kidney. Am J Transplant 2017; 17 (Suppl. 1): 21-116.

[http://dx.doi.org/10.1111/ajt.14124] [PMID: 28052609]

[7]   Rege A, Irish B, Castleberry A, *et al.* Trends in usage and outcomes for expanded criteria donor kidney transplantation in the united states characterized by kidney donor profile index. Cureus 2016; 8(11): e887.
[http://dx.doi.org/10.7759/cureus.887] [PMID: 28018757]

[8]   Latchana N, Peck JR, Whitson BA, Henry ML, Elkhammas EA, Black SM. Preservation solutions used during abdominal transplantation: Current status and outcomes. World J Transplant 2015; 5(4): 154-64.
[http://dx.doi.org/10.5500/wjt.v5.i4.154] [PMID: 26722644]

[9]   Moers C, Smits JM, Maathuis MH, *et al.* Machine perfusion or cold storage in deceased-donor kidney transplantation. N Engl J Med 2009; 360(1): 7-19.
[http://dx.doi.org/10.1056/NEJMoa0802289] [PMID: 19118301]

[10]   Moers C, Pirenne J, Paul A, Ploeg RJ. Machine perfusion or cold storage in deceased-donor kidney transplantation. N Engl J Med 2012; 366(8): 770-1.
[http://dx.doi.org/10.1056/NEJMc1111038] [PMID: 22356343]

[11]   Cannon RM, Brock GN, Garrison RN, Marvin MR, Franklin GA, Davis EG. Machine perfusion: not just for marginal kidney donors. Am Surg 2015; 81(6): 550-6.
[PMID: 26031265]

[12]   Jiao B, Liu S, Liu H, Cheng D, Cheng Y, Liu Y. Hypothermic machine perfusion reduces delayed graft function and improves one-year graft survival of kidneys from expanded criteria donors: a meta-analysis. PLoS One 2013; 8(12): e81826.
[http://dx.doi.org/10.1371/journal.pone.0081826] [PMID: 24339970]

[13]   Shapiro AM, Lakey JR, Ryan EA, *et al.* Islet transplantation in seven patients with type 1 diabetes mellitus using a glucocorticoid-free immunosuppressive regimen. N Engl J Med 2000; 343(4): 230-8.
[http://dx.doi.org/10.1056/NEJM200007273430401] [PMID: 10911004]

CHAPTER 11

Living Donation

Benjamin Philosophe¹, Jaime Glorioso¹, Shane Ottmann¹, Iyore James¹ and **Amer Rajab*, ²**

¹ *Johns Hopkins University School of Medicine, Baltimore, MD, USA*

² *The Ohio State University, Columbus, OH, USA*

Abstract: Living Donation of kidneys and liver has been an important component of organ donation since the field's inception. Living donation requires meticulous examination of potential donors, both to ensure the safety of the donor and assure that the organ is well suited to the recipient. These procedures must be done in a safe and highly reliable way to avoid short and long term complications for the donor. In this chapter, we review specific nuances and recovery techniques in living liver and living kidney donation procedures.

Keywords: Living Donation, Living Donor Kidney Transplantation, Living Donor Liver Transplantation.

INTRODUCTION

Living Donor Liver Transplantation (LDLT)

Living donor liver transplantation (LDLT) for pediatric recipients was introduced in 1989 to overcome the severe shortage of deceased donor organs across the world [1]. In 1993, Tanaka *et al.* reported the first adult-to-adult right liver LDLT using a right lobe, making liver transplantation feasible for adults in areas of the world where deceased donors are very limited [2]. Since then, living donor grafts for adults have expanded to include right lobes with the middle hepatic vein and left lobes. The centers embarking on LDLT often face ethical issues regarding donor safety when a healthy adult must undergo a complicated major surgery without receiving any health benefit. The complication rate after LDLT ranges widely in the literature between 10% and 50% depending on the severity. Unfortunately, there have been a number of deaths after living donation. The risk of death is estimated to be 0.2% to 0.5% with left lobe donation and 0.3% to 1% with right lobe donation. Because of this as well as a highly publicized death of a

---

* **Corresponding author Amer Rajab:** The Ohio State University, Columbus, OH, USA Tel: 614-293-6322; Fax: 614-293-4541; Email: amer.rajab@osumc.edu

Robert S.D. Higgins & Juan A. Sanchez (Eds.)

living donor in New York City, enthusiasm in the United States has waned since 2001, despite a flat number of deceased donor liver transplants in the past 10 years. Five-year survival for living donor liver transplants is around 80%, equal to deceased donor transplants.

Patient Selection

- Living donors should meet the general criteria:
- Have an important personal relationship with the recipient
- Willingly come forward to donate
- Be between the ages of 18 and 60
- Have a compatible blood type with the recipient
- Be in excellent health
- Have a BMI less than 35
- Not have uncontrolled high blood pressure, liver disease, diabetes or heart disease

If these general criteria are met, more specific tests are then performed:

- CXR on all
- Pulmonary Function Tests if history of smoking or asthma
- ECG
- Echocardiogram
- Stress test on donors >50 yo or with significant family history
- Colonoscopy for patients older than 50 yo
- Pap smear/mammograms for females older than 40
- Urinalysis assessing hematuria, proteinuria, micro albumin
- Liver biopsy if possibility of liver disease or steatosis
- Cancer screening including PSA, CEA, AFP, CA 19-9, CA 125
- Laboratory studies including CBC, CMP, Lipid profile, Transferrin, Ferritin, ceruloplasmin, alpha 1-antitrypsin, ANA, AMA, SMA
- Coagulation profile including AntiTIII, APL Ab, Prot C/S, Fact V ligand, vWFa, Fibrinogen, PT G20210 mutation
- Serologies including CMV, HSV, EBV, HBVsAb HBVsAg, HBVcAb, HCVAb/NAT, HIV Ab/NAT, VDRL
- Tissue Typing

Once the donors pass the screening evaluation and tests listed above, they undergo imaging with includes a CT scan, an MRI, MRCP, or a combination. In our institution, we use a triple phase CT scan and an MRCP. MeVis© 3D reconstruction uses both the CT and MRCP to assess liver volume, intended graft volume, venous anatomy and drainage territories, as well as portal venous, biliary and arterial anatomy (Fig. **11.1**).

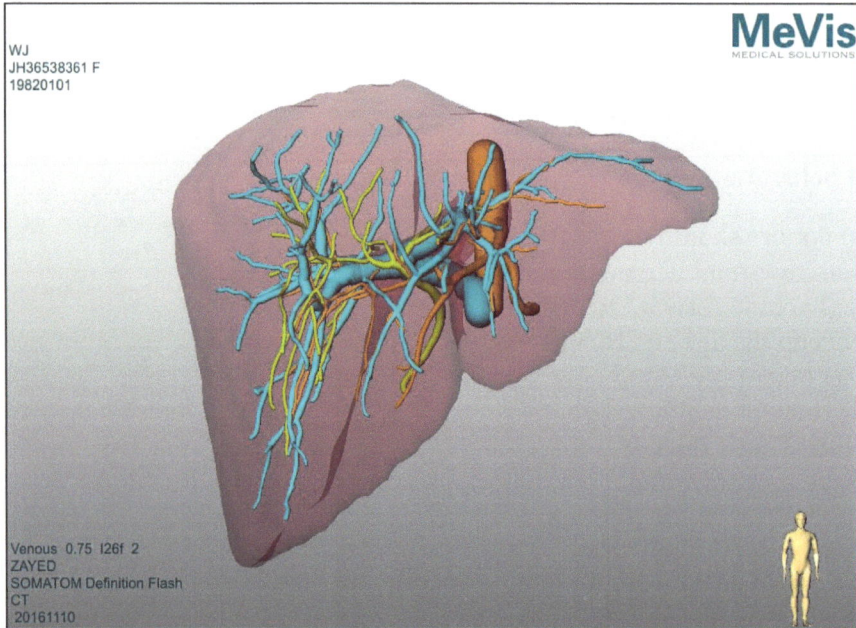

Fig. (11.1). 3D reconstruction of the portal venous, hepatic artery and biliary anatomy. The reconstruction is performed using a three-phase contrast CT and an MRCP. Used with permission. Medical Illustrations© 2018 Tim Phelps, MS, FAMI, Johns Hopkins University.

A multi-disciplinary team evaluates all donors at this point. The team includes a surgeon, hepatologist, nutritionist, pharmacist, nurse or nurse practitioner, and social worker. The psychosocial assessment is an important component of the donor evaluation. All members of the multi-disciplinary team represent the donor and are not involved with the recipient workup.

Graft function following live donor liver transplantation is highly dependent on graft volume. Although left lobe donation is associated with a lower mortality rate, left lobe volumes are typically smaller and small for size syndrome is more prevalent, especially in the face of significant portal hypertension. As a result, right lobe grafts have been used more commonly in adults. Previous literature has suggested that a graft weight/recipient weight ration ≥ 0.8% and a graft weight/standard liver volume ratio of 40% are the same limits for donor graft size to avoid small for size syndrome. Small for size syndrome is defined as prolonged cholestasis with ascites void of technical issues. Imaging techniques to predict vascular anatomy and graft weight include MRIs with iv contrast and or fine cut CT scans with iv contrast. There are multiple software companies that reconstruct the CT or MRI images in 3D to allow the surgeon to more precisely assess graft volume including segmental drainage of the liver. These 3D analyses enable the surgical team to better plan resection lines and need for venous reconstruction.

Parenchymal transection for right lobe grafts is typically performed immediately to the right of the middle hepatic vein. Large branches from segment 5 or 8 draining to the middle hepatic vein may need to be reconstructed to avoid hepatic congestion.

Biliary complications have been the Achilles heel of live donor liver transplants. Biliary anatomy is highly variable and the need to anastomose two bile ducts is not uncommon. As a result, the leak and stricture rate can be as high as 30%, higher than for deceased donor transplants. Despite the technical challenges and higher graft complications, living donor liver transplantation remains a life-saving procedure for patients with end-stage liver disease

There are 2 important parameters to consider when assessing a living donor graft:

1. The graft volume should be assessed not only in the relation to the patient's weight, but the degree of portal hypertension.
2. The residual volume should be ≥30%. Small for size graft occurs more frequently in the setting of significant portal hypertension. The donor graft: recipient weight should be ≥ 0.8%.

The liver anatomy depicted in Fig. (**11.1**), is normal and both left or right grafts would be feasible technically. If the recipient weighs 100 kg for example, a left lobe graft estimated at 483 cc would be too small. Liver density is around 1.05 g/ml, so 483 cc would equal 507 g, which would place the graft to weight ratio at 0.5%. The right lobe graft estimated at 1200 cc would be more appropriate since the graft to weight ratio would be 1.26%. The remnant with a right lobe graft would be an acceptable 30%. If on the other hand the recipient was small and weighed only 50 kg, the left lobe graft would be more appropriate with a graft to recipient weight of 1.0%. Left lobe grafts tend to be safer for donors and should be used for smaller recipients without significant portal hypertension.

Surgical Technique

Donor Right Lobe Hepatectomy

The donor's abdomen is opened with a right subcostal incision with a vertical extension to the xiphoid (Fig. **11.2**). The falciform ligament is divided up to the diaphragm allowing the exposure of the anterior suprahepatic vena cava. The sulcus between the right and middle hepatic veins is clearly defined by clearing the surrounding connective tissue. The left triangular ligament is kept intact to prevent torqueing of the remaining left lobe post donation, which can lead to outflow occlusion and liver failure.

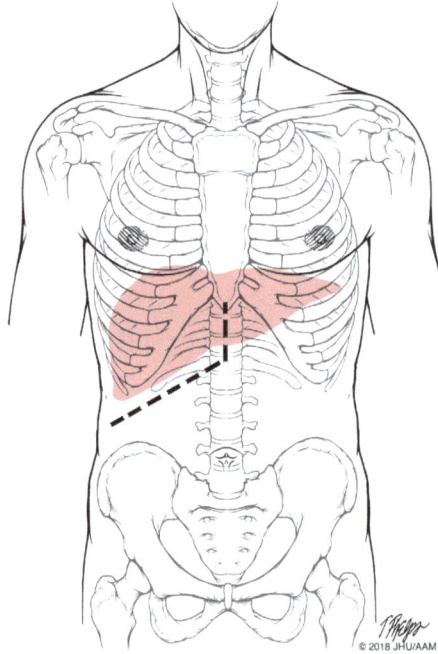

Fig. (11.2). The donor's abdomen is opened with a right subcostal incision with a vertical extension to the xiphoid. Medical Illustrations© 2018 Tim Phelps, MS, FAMI, Johns Hopkins University.

After a cholecystectomy, we routinely perform an intraoperative cholangiogram to confirm the biliary anatomy seen on MRCP. The estimated bile duct bifurcation is tagged with a clip and identified on the Cholangiogram. Aberrant right ducts that drain into the main left duct occur about 10% of the time, and the ones missed on MRCP are identified at this point.

After the cholangiogram, the right hepatic artery is dissected out in its entirety. It often crosses posterior to the common hepatic duct and is usually divided to the left of it. Elevation of the right hepatic artery often exposes the main portal vein. This is dissected proximally towards the liver to clearly free up the left and right branches. One cm of the right portal vein needs to be dissected free to allow proper placement of the vascular clamp at the time of excision. It is vital to know where the takeoff of the left portal vein, is as this will delineate the resection margin and the point where the right portal vein is divided. Dissection in the region where the right hepatic artery comes into contact with the bile duct is avoided because this may result in devascularization of the distal right duct and subsequent anastomotic complications.

The right lobe of the liver is then mobilized medially by separating its diaphragmatic attachments and taking down the right triangular and coronary ligaments, thus exposing the retro-hepatic vena cava. The short hepatic veins draining the posterior aspect of the right lobe are then ligated and divided in continuity up to the level of the right hepatic vein and medially 1 cm to the left of the transection line. The right hepatic vein is then encircled with a vessel loop. If an accessory right hepatic vein draining the posterior aspect of the right lobe into the retrohepatic vena cava is greater than 5 mm, it needs to be preserved and implanted in the recipient. This vessel may be contributing significantly to the venous drainage of the right lobe, and division may result in venous congestion after implantation.

Parenchymal transection is performed at a plane determined by intraoperative ultrasound. The most common instrument for transection is an ultrasonic dissector, which is used without any inflow vascular occlusion. Once the hilum is approached another clip is applied at the intended bile duct transection point and confirmed with a cholangiogram. The bile duct is divided sharply with a scalpel, which subsequently facilitates the remainder of the hepatic transection. The bile duct and hilar plate transection is often anxiety producing since small accessory ducts not seen on the cholangiogram can be encountered at this point. These ducts can drain the posterior right lobe or the caudate, and if smaller than one mm can be tied. A caudate duct can also originate from the left crossing the transection plane. Both ends need to be oversewn in this case. Once the bile duct is transected, the parenchymal transection continues in a caudal to cranial direction until the entire parenchyma is divided. This is aided by the "hanging technique" where a Penrose or red rubber catheter is passed between the middle and right hepatic veins and anterior to the vena cava, and then used to suspend the line of transection [3]. It is not uncommon to encounter sizable segment 5 or 8 veins that drain into the middle hepatic vein and need to be preserved and reconstructed (Fig. **11.3**).

When the timing is right, the patient is heparinized, the right hepatic artery is tied on the proximal end and cut, the portal vein is clamped, the right hepatic vein is clamped, and the veins are cut leaving a cuff on each to oversew with prolene. The liver is extracted and flushed on ice in the backtable with histidine-tryptophan-ketoglutarate (HTK) solution. Both the artery and portal vein are flushed with several hundred cc' until the effluent is clear. Venous reconstruction of segment 5 or 8 veins is done on the backtable using either preserved allograft iliac vein or cryopreserved vessels.

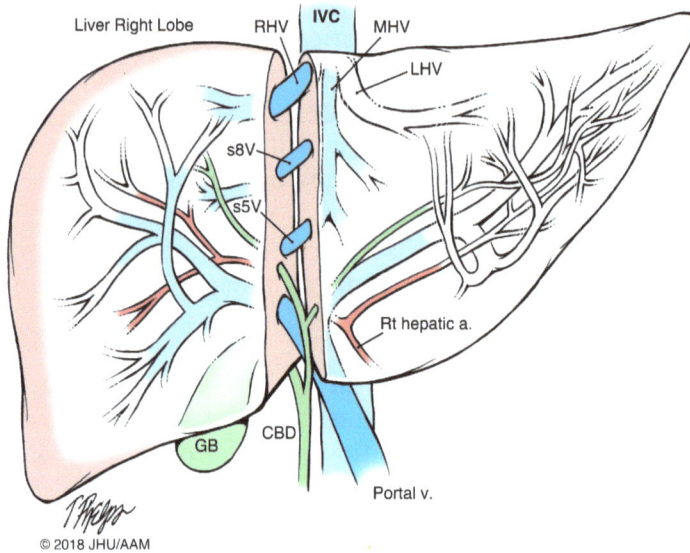

Fig. (11.3). Right hepatic parenchymal dissection and transection. Medical Illustrations© 2018 Tim Phelps, MS, FAMI, Johns Hopkins University.

Donor Left Lobe Hepatectomy

The donor's abdomen is opened with a right subcostal incision with midline vertical extension to the xiphoid process (Fig. **11.2**). The falciform ligament is divided to the level of the diaphragm allowing the exposure of the anterior suprahepatic vena cava. A self-retaining retractor system is placed. The liver is inspected for size and quality. A cholecystectomy is performed; the cystic duct is cannulated and an intraoperative cholangiogram is performed to evaluate the biliary tree and accurately identify the point of transection of the left bile duct. Upon clear visualization of the biliary tree, a vascular clamp is placed at the intended site of dissection and repeat cholangiogram is performed until the desired point for safe bile duct division is achieved.

The hilum is then dissected identifying the left hepatic artery (LHA) and carefully dissecting to the junction with the main hepatic artery (MHA). It is important to avoid injuring segment 4 artery which may arise from the LHA at any level. Upon completely dissecting the LHA, the left portal vein (LPV) is dissected. Small caudate lobe branches originating from the LPV should be double ligated and divided. The caudate lobe branches that are directly connected to the LPV should be left intact. The lesser sac is entered and divided to the level of the diaphragm with care taken not to injure any replaced or accessory LHA. The left lobe of the liver is then mobilized by dividing the left triangular ligament with care taken not to injure the diaphragmatic vein that drains into the left hepatic vein. If necessary, the diaphragmatic vein can be ligated and divided to gain better exposure of the left hepatic vein. The caudate lobe is then mobilized from the inferior vena cava (IVC) ensuring that small hepatic veins that drain directly to the IVC are double ligated and divided. A large hepatic vein should be preserved and anastomosed to IVC to avoid congestion of the caudate lobe. The ductus venosum is dissected and ligated to expose the lateral part of the left hepatic vein. The left hepatic vein (LHV) and middle hepatic vein (MHV) are dissected free from surrounding tissue. The junction of the MHV and right hepatic vein (RHV) is identified. The parenchymal transection line is then identified by temporarily clamping of the LPV and LHA. With an ultrasonic dissector, the parenchyma is transected along the demarcation line. The MHV is included with the graft. Branches of segments 5 and 8 that drained into the MHV should be double ligated to prevent bleeding. Upon reaching the hilar plate, the bile duct is divided with a scalpel. Any bleeding from the biliary duct vessel is controlled with 6-0 PDS sutures. The biliary duct stump is oversewn with running 6-0 PDS sutures.

Once the parenchyma transection is complete (Fig. **11.4**), the LHA and LPV are clamped on the donor graft side. The stump toward to right liver lobe is ligated. The vessels are sharply divided. The common stump of the MHV and LHV is clamped toward the IVC and sharply divided.

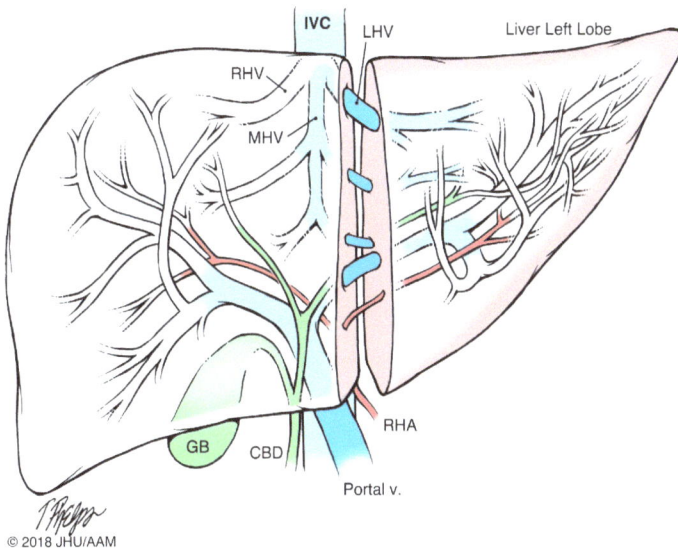

Fig. (11.4). Completed parenchyma transection. Medical Illustrations© 2018 Tim Phelps, MS, FAMI, Johns Hopkins University.

The liver is then transferred to the back table to a basin containing ice sludge. The graft is flushed with histidine-tryptophan-ketoglutarate (HTK) solution. The LHV is cannulated and flushed with at least 1 L of solution. The LHA is cannulated and flushed with 500mL of solution or until the effluent is clear. The common stump of the MHV and LHV is closed with 3-0 Prolene suture in a running fashion. The cut surface of the remnant liver is carefully inspected for bleeding and bile leak. A repeat cholangiogram is performed to ensure no biliary duct injuries or leaks. The donor is carefully inspected to identify any areas of bleeding or bile leak. If the bile leak is found, it is sutured with 6-0 PDS suture. The abdomen is irrigated and closed in 2 layers.

Implantation of the right lobe graft can involve 3 hepatic veins. The main right hepatic vein is anastomosed to the native right hepatic vein orifice that is extended inferiorly along the vena cava. Segment 8 and segment 5 veins that are draining significant portions of the right lobe graft are usually anastomosed directly into the vena cava with separate incisions (Fig. **11.5**).

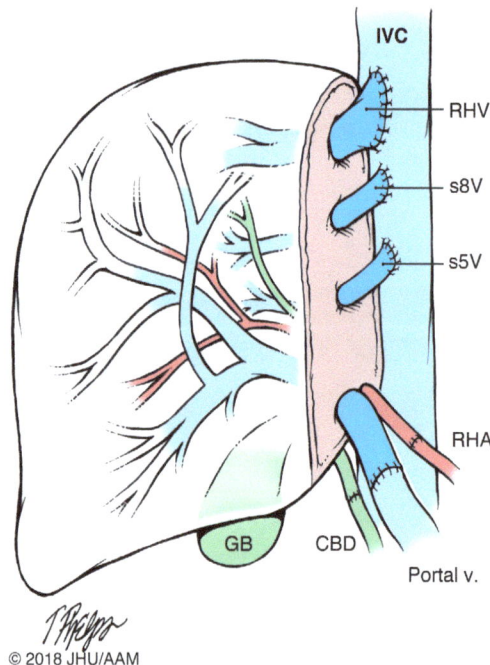

Fig. (11.5). The main right hepatic vein is anastomosed to the native right hepatic vein orifice that is extended inferiorly along the vena cava. Medical Illustrations© 2018 Tim Phelps, MS, FAMI, Johns Hopkins University.

Donor Left Lateral Hepatectomy

Left lateral donor hepatectomy include segments 2 and 3 with or without a portion of segment 4 depending on the size of the recipient. The procedure begins by exposure of the liver *via* a right subcostal incision with midline vertical extension to the xiphoid process. If the donor is thin, an upper midline incision can be used. The falciform ligament is divided to the level of the diaphragm allowing exposure of the anterior suprahepatic vena cava. A self-retaining retractor system is placed. The liver is inspected for size and quality. An intraoperative ultrasonography is performed to delineate the anatomy of segments 2 through 4 and the hepatic veins. The lesser sac is opened and palpated for presence of an accessory or replaced left hepatic artery. If a replaced left hepatic artery is identified, this should be preserved with the graft. A cholecystectomy is performed followed by an intraoperative cholangiogram through the cystic duct stump to identify any biliary anatomic variations. The left triangular ligament is divided. The suprahepatic inferior vena cava is dissected free to expose the common trunk of the left hepatic vein (LHV) and the middle hepatic vein (MHV) with its junction to the inferior vena cava (IVC).

Hilar dissection is then conducted, identifying and isolating the left hepatic artery (LHA) and left portal vein (LPV). Small hepatic veins from the caudate lobe should be recognized and double ligated during dissection of the LPV. The ductus venosum is dissected and ligated at its junction with the IVC to expose the lateral wall of the LHV. The position of the junction of the LHV and MHV should be noted. If the junction is extrahepatic, gentle dissection is carried out around the LHV and extended cephalad to create a plane between the LHV and MHV. The LHV can then be encircled with a vessel loop. However, isolation of the LHV with a vessel loop should not be conducted if the junction of the LHV and MHV is intrahepatic to avoid severe bleeding.

The plane of transection is marked on the anterior surface of the liver with cautery. The transection line should be to the left of the falciform ligament. Parenchymal transection is performed with an ultrasonic dissector starting closer to the hilar plate. Once the hilar plate is reached, a repeat cholangiogram may be performed to confirm the exact point of left hepatic duct division. Once the point of division is identified, the hilar plate along with the left hepatic duct is sharply divided with a scalpel. Bleeding should be controlled with 6-0 PDS suture. Inspect for bile leak; suture ligate if present. Continue parenchyma transection cephalad to the junction of the MHV and LHV. If a large segment IV hepatic vein is encountered, it should be suture ligated to facilitate completion of the hepatectomy. If the recipient needs a portion of segment 4 parenchyma, the transection plane should be moved toward the mid-plane of the liver. If the MHV is encountered, it should be traced to the junction with the LHV and the parenchymal transection plane should be shifted horizontally toward the ductus venosum.

The next step after completion of the parenchymal transection is division of the vessels. The LHA and LPV are separated from the main hepatic artery and main portal vein respectively. The LHV is divided with a vascular stapler.

The liver is then transferred to the back table to a basin containing ice sludge. The graft is flushed with histidine-tryptophan-ketoglutarate (HTK) solution. The LHV is cannulated and flushed with at least 1 L of solution. The LHA is cannulated and flushed with 500mL of solution or until the effluent is clear. The donor is carefully inspected to identify any areas of bleeding or bile leak. If the bile leak is found, it is sutured with 6-0 PDS suture. The abdomen is irrigated and closed in 2 layers.

LIVING DONATION- KIDNEY

Introduction

The number of individuals with end stage renal disease awaiting kidney transplantation continues to rise. In the United States, there are more than 95,000 patients on the kidney transplant waiting list [4]. Living donor kidney transplant significantly benefits patients with end stage renal disease and is one approach to both decrease the number of patients awaiting transplantation and wait list time. As the gap between the number of patients awaiting kidney transplant and the number of deceased donors widens, increased pressure is placed on transplant centers to consider living donors with more complex medical conditions. This chapter will emphasize the evaluation of the living kidney donor, as minimizing risk to the living donor is of the upmost importance.

The first successful living donor kidney transplant took place in Boston in 1954 by the pioneering surgeon, Dr. Joseph Murray [5]. Ronald Herrick donated a kidney to his monozygotic twin, Richard, who was suffering from end stage renal disease. The donor nephrectomy was uncomplicated. The recipient lived 56 years' post-transplant and represents the first transplant to result in long term success. This altruistic gift set in motion a multitude of advances in the field of transplantation worldwide.

Since the first living donor kidney transplant over 60 years ago, the popularity of living donor kidney donation has waxed and waned. With the establishment of brain death criteria in the 1970s and the improvement in immunosuppressant medications in the 1980s, deceased donor kidney transplantation predominated.

However, living donation increased 30-40% annually early in the decade and by 1989 accounted for 21% of all kidney transplants [6]. The last decade of the twentieth century brought escalating interest in living donor kidney transplantation secondary to extended wait list times and the introduction of laparoscopic surgery. Minimally invasive techniques result in comparable outcomes with the benefit of improved postoperative pain, shorter hospitalization, and faster recovery [7, 8]. Currently, living donation accounts for approximately 38% of all kidney transplants in the United States [4]. At the peak in 2004, 6,436 individuals (51% of kidney transplants in the United States) received a living donor kidney transplant [9]. Since that time, the percentage of living donation has declined, in part due to the rise in the absolute number of deceased donor kidney transplant. The number of related living donation has decreased despite an increase in the number of non-related kidney donors.

Benefits of Living Donor Kidney Transplant

Patients receiving allografts from a living donor benefit from improved graft and overall survival compared to deceased donor kidney transplant recipients. Improved graft survival subsequently leads to lower rates of re-transplants and fewer patients re-entering the waitlist. Recipients of a living donor kidney experience shorter waiting times. Living donor transplantation is the only option for undergoing transplantation prior to the initiation of dialysis, which has been shown to be beneficial in terms of graft survival [10]. Kidneys from deceased donors have higher rates of primary non function and delayed graft function when compared to living donor kidneys. With the convenience of scheduling, the recipient can be medically optimized for the day of the operation. Finally, living donation allows for kidney exchange programs to better match donor and recipients. Paired kidney donation is a successful strategy for those willing to donate but have ABO or HLA incompatibility with their intended recipient and therefore increases the donor pool.

Donor Evaluation

The evaluated of a living donor candidate should confirm the individual in good health, has normal renal function and structure, and is not a risk to the recipient with respect to transmission of malignancy or infection. Most importantly, the evaluation determines potential risk to the donor as a consequence of donation. Guidelines have been set forth for evaluation of living donor candidates to establish consistent and thorough evaluations across transplant centers. The Organ Procurement and Transplantation Network (OPTN) Living Donor policy statement, initially implemented in 2013, provides requirements pertaining to informed consent, psychosocial evaluation, medical evaluation, and post-donation follow up [11]. This statement along with recent clinical guidelines from the KDIGO Living Kidney Donor Work Group [12] and the Amsterdam Forum Guidelines [13] provide the foundation for living kidney donation evaluation.

Broadly speaking, the OPTN guidelines specify that blood typing, a medical evaluation, and a psychological evaluation be completed prior to donation. An Independent Living Donor Advocate (ILDA) must be appointed at all recovering hospitals. This individual will not be involved with the recipient evaluation and acts on the potential donor's behalf, advocating for the rights of the donor [14]. Potential donors will be educated on all phases of the donation process. The donor must be willing to donate, without evidence of coercion. They must be given the opportunity to stop the evaluation process at any point with the understanding that this decision will remain confidential. The surgical, medical, psychosocial and financial risks associated with living donation are discussed in detail with any potential recipient.

Exclusion criteria for living kidney donation, as defined by the OPTN, include: Age <18 years, mental inability to make an informed decision, uncontrolled hypertension or hypertension with evidence of end organ damage, HIV infection, diabetes mellitus, active malignancy, acute infection, uncontrolled psychiatric illness and suspicion of financial or emotional donor coercion [11].

Blood type and crossmatch compatibility should be performed early in the donor assessment. ABO typing should be performed on two separate occasions. The crossmatch between potential donor and recipient is required by UNOS prior to donation and detects preformed antibodies that could cause early allograft failure. Human leukocyte antigen (HLA) testing provides additional prognostic information for graft survival and optimizes matching if there are multiple suitable donors for a recipient. For potential donors that are not biologically compatible, participation in donor change programs can be discussed.

To ensure the potential donor is in good health, a thorough medical evaluation is completed. Refer to Table. **11.1** for evaluation summary. This evaluation includes, but is not limited to, personal medical history of cardiovascular (hypertension, dyslipidemia) and pulmonary risk factors, malignancy, diabetes, hematologic disorders, immunologic disorders, and genitourinary disorders. Kidney specific factors are reviewed and necessitates close attention for related donors when the recipient renal disease is related to a genetic condition. Current and past medications are reviewed. Vital signs, height, weight and BMI are included with the physical exam, with vital sign checks performed over multiple visits. Laboratory testing provides objective data to confirm information obtained from the medical history and identify undiagnosed comorbidities that may preclude donations. The workup includes complete blood count, coagulation studies, a comprehensive metabolic panel and fasting lipid panel for all patients. A chest x-ray and electrocardiogram should be obtained. Premenopausal women should have a quantitative pregnancy test.

Table 11.1. Assessment of kidney donor candidates. (Adapted from: MacConmara MP: Medical Evaluation of the Living Donor. In Kidney Transplantation Principles and Practice Ed. 7th 2014).

Donor Evaluation
History and Physical Exam Complete health questionnaire Detailed history and physical exam by physician Personal or family history of renal disease Active and past medications Family history Vital signs on multiple visits Additional 24 hour blood pressure monitoring, if indicated Height, weight, body mass index Electrocardiogram and chest x-ray
Laboratory Testing ABO blood typing 24 hour urine collection- GFR, urine protein Crossmatch Urinalysis and culture Human leukocyte antigen typing Metabolic panel if history of nephrolithiasis Complete blood count with differential Oral glucose tolerance test and Hemoglobin A1C, if indicated Coagulation studies Human chorionic gonadotropin- quantitative, if indicated Comprehensive metabolic panel Fasting lipid panel
Health Screening **Infection:** HIV Ag/Ab, hepatitis B surface Ag and core Ab, hepatitis C Ab, TB, CMV Ab, EBV Ab, Syphilis Additional testing based on risk factors and geography **Malignancy:** Mammogram, pap smear, prostate exam, prostate specific antigen, colonoscopy, skin exam
Psychosocial Evaluation Complete assessment by psychiatrist, psychologist, or licensed clinical social worker Details social history- occupation, exposure, substance abuse, high risk behaviors Assessment of social support network and coping mechanisms
Imaging CT angiogram or MR angiogram Nuclear medicine study, if indicated
Informed Consent Designated independent living donor advocate Disclosure of short and long term risks of donation Assess ability to provide informed consent Determine decision to donate free from coercion

Donor candidates with BP >140/90 by ambulatory blood pressure monitoring are generally not acceptable donors. Some patients with well-controlled hypertension, who meet other criteria, may be considered but require close follow up postoperatively [15, 16]. Patients with a BMI >35 kg/m^2 should be counselled to lose weight prior to donation. Lifestyle modification education should be provided. If other comorbidities are present, the risk of donation may be too great to proceed. Dyslipidemia should be evaluated in the context of other comorbidities, but alone should not preclude donation. Pulmonary function testing should be utilized selectively for donor candidates with associated risk factors. Individuals with intermediate or major predictors for cardiac complications are excluded from donation. This includes mild angina, previous myocardial infarction, history or presence of heart failure, significant arrhythmias, and severe valvular disease. Cardiac evaluation is indicated for older donors, abnormal electrocardiogram, low cardiac functional capacity, or if warranted based on past medical history. Smoking cessation must be initiated at least four weeks prior to donation and counseling should be provided to promote long term discontinuation of tobacco products.

Patients with a family history or personal history of elevated serum glucose should be evaluated with a glucose tolerance test or hemoglobin A1C. Most practice guidelines strongly recommend against diabetic patients undergoing donor nephrectomy [13, 17]. The recent KDIGO work group recommendations along with several other societies have suggested that patients with type 2 diabetes mellitus may be considered donor candidates, but this must be determined on a case by case basis (KDIGO and European study). Patients with pre-diabetes or risk factors for diabetes also must be carefully selected as type 2 diabetes is the leading cause of chronic kidney disease worldwide and accounts for approximately half of adult onset end stage renal disease [18]. Donors at risk for diabetes should be counselled about their risk for progression to end state renal disease. Younger donors with risk factors are particularly vulnerable [19].

Renal specific investigations include urinalysis with microscopy, urinary protein and albumin excretion and measurement of glomerular filtration rate (GFR). GFR can be measured by creatinine clearance calculated from a 24-hour collection, cystatin C, or by isotopic methods. Hospitals should use the best available method at their institution to estimate GFR. A GFR of at least 80 mL/min/1.73 m^2 has traditionally been the standard cut off for eligibility. However, the KDIGO guidelines recommend a higher threshold value of GRF ($\geq$ 90 mL/min/1.73 m^2) to routinely accept a donor and a lower threshold of GFR <60 mL/min/1.73 m^2 to routinely decline a candidate. For individuals with a GFR between 60-90 mL/min/1.73 m^2, centers can individualize their selection based on comorbidities, age, sex, and other variables. Additional urine studies may be required if the potential donor has a history of nephrolithiasis or evidence of stones on imaging.

Testing for transmissible infectious diseases must include: cytomegalovirus (CMV) antibody, Epstein-Barr virus (EBV) antibody, HIV testing, Hepatitis B surface antigen and core antibody, hepatitis C antibody, and syphilis testing. Further workup will be dictated by the regional risks of transmissible disease and candidate donor travel history. Testing should be completed within four weeks of planned donation.

The OPTN guidelines require appropriate cancer screening be completed prior to donation. This includes age appropriate screening for cervical, breast, prostate, colon, and lung cancer based on recommendations from the American Cancer Society and US Preventative Services Task Force.

A comprehensive psychosocial evaluation is completed by a psychologist, psychiatrist, or licensed clinical social worker. This should include occupation, employment, insurance status, living arrangement, and social support network. Smoking, alcohol, drug use and abuse are reviewed. Screening for high risk behavior should be completed. If high risk behaviors are identified, the potential donor is encouraged to disclose these behaviors to the potential recipient. They should be advised they can withdraw from donation prior to disclosure. The evaluation should also focus on any mental health issues that may result in poor psychosocial outcome following donation and identify any potential factors that may complicate recovery. The donor's ability to cope with the multiple stressor surrounding donation and development of a plan for recovery should be discussed.

The anatomic characteristics of the kidneys are evaluated by imaging, typically CT angiogram or MR angiogram. The imaging protocol should include a non-contrast series to evaluate for nephrolithiasis and vascular calcification along with arterial and venous phases. The kidneys are evaluated for size, evidence of mass, cysts, or stones. The vascular anatomy is reviewed and genitourinary anatomic abnormalities are ruled out. If there is a size discrepancy between the right and left kidney, a nuclear medicine scan may be indicated. If there is functional discrepancy, the higher performing kidney should remain with the donor.

Operative Approach

The donor nephrectomy has evolved over the past several decades with the development of minimally invasive techniques. Today, the vast majority of donor nephrectomies are performed by a minimally invasive technique compared to approximately 45% in 2000 [20]. As previously discussed, the minimally invasive techniques are attractive to potential donors without untoward consequences for the allograft. There is significant practice variability for surgical approach: pure laparoscopic *vs.* hand-assisted *vs.* robotic, laparoscopic *vs.* retroperitoneoscopic, and multiple *vs.* single-site techniques. The benefits to each approach can be debated, but ultimately the technique with which the surgeon is most expertise should be the preferred approach. Left donor nephrectomy is technically easier to perform and yields a graft with a longer renal vein; therefore it is most frequently utilized for living donation.

The key steps of the operation are the same regardless of the approach. For a left, laparoscopic-based approach, after gaining access to the abdomen, the left colon should be mobilized medially along the avascular plane. Gerota's fascia overlying the left renal vein is incised, exposing the gonadal and adrenal veins (Fig. **11.6**). Further dissection of Gerota's fascia laterally along the superior pole of the kidney exposes the adrenal gland. Next, the gonadal vein is followed inferiorly and the ureter is identified and exposed. A window is created in the soft tissue deep to the ureter and extended proximally and distally. The hilar dissection is undertaken next, fully exposing the renal artery and vein. The remaining lateral attachments are divided. Clips are applied to smaller vessels and the ureter. The renal artery and vein are transected with a stapling device preserving as much length as possible. The kidney is extracted through the hand port or a Pfannenstiel incision. The back table flush can be expedited by having the recipient surgeon available. The surgical bed should be inspected to ensure hemostasis.

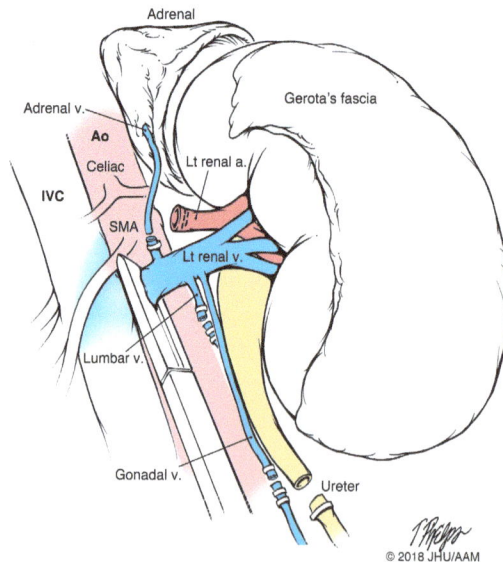

Fig. (11.6). Left kidney with endovascular stapler dividing left renal vein. Medical Illustrations© 2018 Tim Phelps, MS, FAMI, Johns Hopkins University.

Right donor nephrectomy is performed in a similar fashion, with few adjustments to account for the variation in anatomy compared to the left side. An additional port may be required to retract the liver to gain adequate exposure. The right colon and the duodenum will be mobilized medially to expose the renal hilum. As the right renal artery courses posterior to the inferior vena cava, gentle traction on the IVC at the time of arterial transection will increase the length of the allograft artery.

Open donor nephrectomy may be indicated for patients with significant prior abdominal surgery that would preclude a laparoscopic approach or in cases of complex vascular anatomy. Open approaches are performed through a flank incision, utilizing a retroperitoneal approach. A muscle-sparing, mini-open technique minimizes the morbidity of a full flank incision and is comparable to a laparoscopic approach in terms of postoperative pain and allograft function [21].

Complications

Donor nephrectomy is a safe operation with very low risk of complications. However, this must be viewed in the context of placing a healthy individual at such risk, with the wellbeing of the donor seen as a top priority for all transplant center. Any deviation from this tenet puts donor trust in the multidisciplinary team at risk. While complications following donor nephrectomy are infrequent, the potential short and long term ramifications of donation must be discussed in depth with all candidate donors. Perioperative complications include hemorrhage, vascular injury, bowel obstruction, pneumothorax, venous thromboembolism and infectious complications. The risk of death is exceedingly low at 0.02-0.03% and is unchanged over the past two decades [22, 23]. Readmission rate follow donor nephrectomy is approximately 1.5%. A recent study of 97 US centers found an overall donor complication rate of 16.8%. African American donors were more likely to experience a complication (aOR 1.26) compared to Caucasian donors [24]. Increasing age, male sex, obesity were each associated with an increased risk from perioperative complication. Preoperative comorbidities associated with increased complication rates included genitourinary conditions, hematologic disorders, and psychiatric diagnosis. Planned open nephrectomy and robotic nephrectomy also carried higher complications rates compared to a laparoscopic approach. High volume centers (>50 donor nephrectomies annually) predicted lower risk [24].

Potential long term complications following donor nephrectomy include hypertension, gout, metabolic bone, disease, gestational hypertension and ESRD. Several studies comparing rates of ESRD between kidney donors and the general population have found no difference in the rate of ESRD [25, 26]. Long term follow-up is modest. The rate of ESRD after living donation is approximately 0.134 per 1000 years in a study reviewing living donation between 1994 and 2003. Living donors are inherently healthier than the general population due to the rigorous selection process. Therefore, the general population based studies my underestimate to risk of ESRD for donors. Several studies have utilized demographically matched healthy controls and have found a small increased risk of ESRD with donation, although the absolute risk remains quite low [27, 28]. Risk indices have been developed to estimate long term risk of ESRD for donor candidates [29, 30]. Prior living donors receive priority points in the United States kidney allocation system.

The data regarding risk of hypertension following donor nephrectomy is conflicting [31, 32]. A large meta-analysis found an increase in systolic and diastolic blood pressure (6 mmHg and 4 mmHg, respectively) post-donation when compared to controls [33]. A retrospective study demonstrated 40% risk of hypertension among African American donors compared to 18% among matched controlled emphasizing the importance of close follow-up for this at risk population [34].

Women of childbearing age presenting as donor candidates should be informed of the potential risks with pregnancy, specifically gestational hypertension and preeclampsia, following donor nephrectomy [35]. Consensus guidelines require these risks be conveyed to the donor candidate, but plans for future pregnancy should not be a contraindication to donation. Overall, the outcomes of post-donation pregnancies are similar to the general population [36].

Transplant centers carry the responsibility to provide care for the donor beyond the immediate perioperative period. Follow up care in the early postoperative period is universally accepted. However, long term follow-up remains a challenge due to financial and time constraints. The ethical obligation to support the clinical needs for individuals who donate along with the need to acquire data to improve outcomes for future donors outweighs the limitations above [37]. Follow up care should include general health maintenance but focus on kidney health to detect and lifestyle risk factors or new onset comorbidities that would put an individual at increased risk for progressive kidney disease. Furthermore, data suggests up to 25% of kidney donors experience difficulty in obtaining health insurance following donation creating undue stress and potentially limiting follow up secondary to financial concerns [38].

CONCLUDING REMARKS

Living kidney donation clearly benefits individuals with end stage renal disease. A thorough multidisciplinary candidate donor evaluation, excellent perioperative care, and ongoing long term follow up are essential for meeting the primary goal of living donor kidney transplant: optimizing the health and wellbeing of the donor while treating end stage renal disease by providing high quality organs to the recipient. Further research in defining and understanding disparities in living donation as well as gaining further understanding of the long term risks associated with donation need attention.

CONSENT FOR PUBLICATION

Not applicable.

CONFLICT OF INTEREST

The author declares no conflict of interest, financial or otherwise.

ACKNOWLEDGEMENTS

Declared none.

REFERENCES

[1]   Strong RW, Lynch SV, Ong TH, *et al.* Successful liver transplantation from a living donor to her son. NEJM 1990; 24; 322(21): 1505-07.

[2]   Tanaka K, Uemoto S, Tokunaga Y, *et al.* Surgical techniques and innovations in living related liver transplantation. Ann Surg 1993; 217(1): 82-91.
      [http://dx.doi.org/10.1097/00000658-199301000-00014] [PMID: 8424706]

[3]   Belghiti J, Kianmanesh R. Surgical techniques used in adult living donor liver transplantation. Liver Transpl 2003; 9(10) (Suppl. 2): S29-34.
      [http://dx.doi.org/10.1053/jlts.2003.50226] [PMID: 14528425]

[4]   Organ procurement and Transplant Network (OPTN) National data reports, transplants by donor type, latest data. [cited: August 1, 2017] Available from: https://www.unos.org/data/transplant-trends/ #waitlists_by_organ

[5]   Murray JE. Ronald Lee Herrick Memorial: June 15, 1931-December 27, 2010. Am J Transplant 2011; 11(3): 419.
      [http://dx.doi.org/10.1111/j.1600-6143.2011.03445.x] [PMID: 21342441]

[6]   Bertolatus JA. Renal Transplantation for the nephrologist: living donor kidney transplantation: what did we learn from the 1980s? Am J Kidney Dis 1991; 17(5): 596-9.
      [http://dx.doi.org/10.1016/S0272-6386(12)80505-1] [PMID: 2024664]

[7]   Ratner LE, Kavoussi LR, Sroka M, *et al.* Laparoscopic assisted live donor nephrectomy--a comparison with the open approach. Transplantation 1997; 63(2): 229-33.
      [http://dx.doi.org/10.1097/00007890-199701270-00009] [PMID: 9020322]

[8]   Yuan H, Liu L, Zheng S, *et al.* The safety and efficacy of laparoscopic donor nephrectomy for renal transplantation: an updated meta-analysis. Transplant Proc 2013; 45(1): 65-76.
      [http://dx.doi.org/10.1016/j.transproceed.2012.07.152] [PMID: 23375276]

[9]   OPTN (Organ Procurement and Transplantation Network)/UNOS (United Network for Organ Sharing) National data Reports. [cited: August 1, 2017] Available from: http://optn.transplant.hrsa.gov/ data/view-data-report/national-data/

[10]   Meier-Kriesche HU, Kaplan B. Waiting time on dialysis as the strongest modifiable risk factor for renal transplant outcomes: a paired donor kidney analysis. Transplantation 2002; 74(10): 1377-81.
[http://dx.doi.org/10.1097/00007890-200211270-00005] [PMID: 12451234]

[11]   Meier-Kriesche HU, Kaplan B. Waiting time on dialysis as the strongest modifiable risk factor for renal transplant outcomes: a paired donor kidney analysis. Transplantation 2002; 74(10): 1377-81.
[http://dx.doi.org/10.1097/00007890-200211270-00005] [PMID: 12451234]

[12]   Kidney Disease: Improving Global Outcomes (KDIGO) Living Kidney Donor Work Group. KDIGO clinical practice guideline on the evaluation and care of living kidney donors. Transplantation 2017; 101 (Suppl. 8S): S1-S109.

[13]   Delmonico F. A report of the Amsterdam Forum on the care of the live kidney donor: data and medical guidelines. Transplantation 2005; 79(6) (Suppl.): S53-66.
[PMID: 15785361]

[14]   Hays RE, LaPointe Rudow D, Dew MA, Taler SJ, Spicer H, Mandelbrot DA. The independent living donor advocate: a guidance document from the American Society of Transplantation's Living Donor Community of Practice (AST LDCOP). Am J Transplant 2015; 15(2): 518-25.
[http://dx.doi.org/10.1111/ajt.13001] [PMID: 25612499]

[15]   Textor SC, Taler SJ, Driscoll N, *et al.* Blood pressure and renal function after kidney donation from hypertensive living donors. Transplantation 2004; 78(2): 276-82.
[http://dx.doi.org/10.1097/01.TP.0000128168.97735.B3] [PMID: 15280690]

[16]   Tent H, Sanders JS, Rook M, *et al.* Effects of preexistent hypertension on blood pressure and residual renal function after donor nephrectomy. Transplantation 2012; 93(4): 412-7.
[http://dx.doi.org/10.1097/TP.0b013e318240e9b9] [PMID: 22217533]

[17]   Pascual J, Abramowicz D, Cochat P, *et al.* European renal best practice guideline on the management and evaluation of the kidney donor and recipient. Nefrologia 2014; 34(3): 293-301.
[PMID: 24798566]

[18]   Narayan KM, Boyle JP, Thompson TJ, Sorensen SW, Williamson DF. Lifetime risk for diabetes mellitus in the United States. JAMA 2003; 290(14): 1884-90.
[http://dx.doi.org/10.1001/jama.290.14.1884] [PMID: 14532317]

[19]   Ligthart S, van Herpt TT, Leening MJ, *et al.* Lifetime risk of developing impaired glucose metabolism and eventual progression from prediabetes to type 2 diabetes: a prospective cohort study. Lancet Diabetes Endocrinol 2016; 4(1): 44-51.
[http://dx.doi.org/10.1016/S2213-8587(15)00362-9] [PMID: 26575606]

[20]   Troppmann C, Ormond DB, Perez RV. Laparoscopic (vs open) live donor nephrectomy: a UNOS database analysis of early graft function and survival. Am J Transplant 2003; 3(10): 1295-301.
[http://dx.doi.org/10.1046/j.1600-6143.2003.00216.x] [PMID: 14510704]

[21]   Yadav K, Aggarwal S, Guleria S, Kumar R. Comparative study of laparoscopic and mini-incision open donor nephrectomy: have we heard the last word in the debate? Clin Transplant 2016; 30(3): 328-34.
[http://dx.doi.org/10.1111/ctr.12700] [PMID: 26780835]

[22]   Segev DL, Muzaale AD, Caffo BS, *et al.* Perioperative mortality and long-term survival following live kidney donation. JAMA 2010; 303(10): 959-66.
[http://dx.doi.org/10.1001/jama.2010.237] [PMID: 20215610]

[23]   Matas AJ, Bartlett ST, Leichtman AB, Delmonico FL. Morbidity and mortality after living kidney donation, 1999-2001: survey of United States transplant centers. Am J Transplant 2003; 3(7): 830-4.
[PMID: 12814474]

[24]   Lentine KL, Lam NN, Axelrod D, *et al.* Perioperative complications after living kidney donation: A national study. Am J Transplant 2016; 16(6): 1848-57.
[http://dx.doi.org/10.1111/ajt.13687] [PMID: 26700551]

[25]   Fehrman-Ekholm I, Dunér F, Brink B, Tydén G, Elinder CG. No evidence of accelerated loss of kidney function in living kidney donors: results from a cross-sectional follow-up. Transplantation 2001; 72(3): 444-9.
[http://dx.doi.org/10.1097/00007890-200108150-00015] [PMID: 11502974]

[26]   Mjøen G, Hallan S, Hartmann A, *et al.* Long-term risks for kidney donors. Kidney Int 2014; 86(1): 162-7.
[http://dx.doi.org/10.1038/ki.2013.460] [PMID: 24284516]

[27]   Cherikh WS, Young CJ, Kramer BF, Taranto SE, Randall HB, Fan PY. Ethnic and gender related differences in the risk of end-stage renal disease after living kidney donation. Am J Transplant 2011; 11(8): 1650-5.
[http://dx.doi.org/10.1111/j.1600-6143.2011.03609.x] [PMID: 21672160]

[28]   Muzaale AD, Massie AB, Wang MC, *et al.* Risk of end-stage renal disease following live kidney donation. JAMA 2014; 311(6): 579-86.
[http://dx.doi.org/10.1001/jama.2013.285141] [PMID: 24519297]

[29]   Massie AB, Leanza J, Fahmy LM, *et al.* A risk index for living donor kidney transplantation. Am J Transplant 2016; 16(7): 2077-84.
[http://dx.doi.org/10.1111/ajt.13709] [PMID: 26752290]

[30]   Grams ME, Sang Y, Levey AS, *et al.* Kidney-failure risk projection for the living kidney-donor candidate. N Engl J Med 2016; 374(5): 411-21.
[http://dx.doi.org/10.1056/NEJMoa1510491] [PMID: 26544982]

[31]   Kasiske BL, Anderson-Haag T, Israni AK, *et al.* A prospective controlled study of living kidney donors: three-year follow-up. Am J Kidney Dis 2015; 66(1): 114-24.
[http://dx.doi.org/10.1053/j.ajkd.2015.01.019] [PMID: 25795073]

[32]   Garg AX, Prasad GV, Thiessen-Philbrook HR, *et al.* Cardiovascular disease and hypertension risk in living kidney donors: an analysis of health administrative data in Ontario, Canada. Transplantation 2008; 86(3): 399-406.
[http://dx.doi.org/10.1097/TP.0b013e31817ba9e3] [PMID: 18698242]

[33]   Boudville N, Prasad GV, Knoll G, *et al.* Meta-analysis: risk for hypertension in living kidney donors. Ann Intern Med 2006; 145(3): 185-96.
[http://dx.doi.org/10.7326/0003-4819-145-3-200608010-00006] [PMID: 16880460]

[34]   Doshi MD, Goggins MO, Li L, Garg AX. Medical outcomes in African American live kidney donors: a matched cohort study. Am J Transplant 2013; 13(1): 111-8.
[http://dx.doi.org/10.1111/j.1600-6143.2012.04303.x] [PMID: 23094818]

[35]   Ibrahim HN, Akkina SK, Leister E, *et al.* Pregnancy outcomes after kidney donation. Am J Transplant 2009; 9(4): 825-34.
[http://dx.doi.org/10.1111/j.1600-6143.2009.02548.x] [PMID: 19353771]

[36]   Garg AX, Nevis IF, McArthur E, *et al.* Gestational hypertension and preeclampsia in living kidney donors. N Engl J Med 2015; 372(2): 124-33.
[http://dx.doi.org/10.1056/NEJMoa1408932] [PMID: 25397608]

[37]   Leichtman A, Abecassis M, Barr M, *et al.* Living kidney donor follow-up: state-of-the-art and future directions, conference summary and recommendations. Am J Transplant 2011; 11(12): 2561-8.
[http://dx.doi.org/10.1111/j.1600-6143.2011.03816.x] [PMID: 22054039]

[38]   Boyarsky BJ, Massie AB, Alejo JL, *et al.* Experiences obtaining insurance after live kidney donation. Am J Transplant 2014; 14(9): 2168-72.
[http://dx.doi.org/10.1111/ajt.12819] [PMID: 25041695]

CHAPTER 12

Pediatric Issues: Split Liver/Living Liver Donation

Kyle Jackson, Benjamin Philosophe and Andrew Cameron[*]

Johns Hopkins University School of Medicine, Baltimore, MD, USA

Abstract: In this chapter, we review the technical nuances and donor-recipient matching principles of the adult-pediatric split liver donation and living donor transplant process. Specific attention is paid to the safe conduct of the procedures, which in the case of living donation, have high stakes consequences for both the recipient and the donor.

Keywords: Deceased Donor Split Liver Procurement, Living Donor Liver Donation, Pediatric Liver Transplantation, Pediatric Transplantation.

INTRODUCTION

Liver transplantation continues to be the only curative therapy for pediatric (age < 18 years) patients with irreversible acute or chronic end-stage liver disease. Long-term outcomes following pediatric liver transplantation (PLT) are generally excellent, with one-year and long-term patient survival exceeding 90% and 80%, respectively [1 - 3]. Indications for liver transplantation in the pediatric population differ significantly from those in adults. Biliary atresia, a cholestatic disorder, represents the primary indication for PLT, accounting for over 40% of all PLT [4]. Beyond survival, the majority of PLT recipients lead normal lives. As many as 80% attend normal school, and 70% do so without any kind of performance delay [5]. With excellent long-term survival and functional outcomes following PLT, it is critical to ensure that every child in need of liver transplantation receives it. However, as with adult transplantation, there continues to be a scarcity of donor organs.

Nationally, there is a large discrepancy between the number of patients awaiting liver transplantation and the number of donor organs available. In 2016, 573 children received a liver transplant [6]. Despite this, as of August 2017, approximately 469 children remain on the waiting list for liver transplantation, with new potential recipients being added to the list daily [6]. A number of

[*] **Corresponding author Andrew Cameron:** Johns Hopkins University School of Medicine, Baltimore, MD, USA; Tel: 410502-5198; Fax: 410510-1514; Email: acamero5@jhmi.edu

Robert S.D. Higgins & Juan A. Sanchez (Eds.)

different policies and practices have been adopted to attempt to increase the donor pool to meet the ever-increasing need for liver transplantation, with varying degrees of success [7 - 9]. Examples of such practices include the development of the Share-35 allocation policy, the use of donors following cardiac death, the use of livers from donors with human immunodeficiency virus, the use of split livers, and increasing the amount of living donors utilized. We will focus here on the latter two: using split livers and living donor liver transplantation.

SPLIT LIVER TRANSPLANTATION

Introduction

Split liver transplantation (SLT) is a technique that has been developed to help increase the availability of liver grafts for both adult and pediatric recipients. Using this technique, a donor liver is "split" into two smaller grafts, generally with one larger than the other. The smaller graft is usually given to a pediatric recipient, whereas the larger is given to the adult recipient. By creating two grafts from one donor liver, SLT allows two recipients to receive a liver transplant from a single donor, thereby increasing the number of patients who benefit from a scarce resource.

The technique was first attempted in 1988, but was considered risky and experimental for many years following [10]. To be sure, initial results were poor, due to a combination of inexperience with the technical aspects and poor donor and recipient selection [11, 12]. However, an increasing number of wait-list deaths in Europe in the early 1990s all but forced some centers there to continue to utilize this technique. By the late-1990s, sufficient experience existed with SLT such that outcomes were good enough to warrant more widespread adoption [13]. As SLT spread, further refinements were made and it has slowly developed into the technique we know it as today.

Technical Aspects

SLT has two major variants, which can be anatomically described using Couinaud's classification of hepatic segments. The first, and more common, variant divides the liver into a left lateral segment (II, III) and a right extended graft (I, IV-VIII). The second divides the liver into two roughly equal hemi-livers (I-IV and V-VIII). While each variant has its own advantages and disadvantages, the flexibility of being able to perform either ensures that the right technique can be used to appropriately match graft volumes to both potential recipients.

Liver splitting can either be done prior to whole liver procurement and infusion of preservative solution ("*in situ*") or on the back table after whole liver procurement ("*ex situ*"). Splitting *in situ* affords better hemostasis of the cut surface of the liver and a better assessment of whether segment IV is ischemic; however, it requires prolonged operative time and a higher degree of hepatobiliary expertise from the procurement team. We describe *in situ* splitting below, but techniques for *ex situ* splitting are not substantially different.

The first variant is the more traditional choice for liver splitting as it provides one larger graft that can be given to an adult, and a smaller graft that can be given to a pediatric recipient. In this form, the left hepatic vein is identified and encircled with a vessel loop. Next, the hepatoduodenal ligament is identified and exposed from left to right, leading to identification of the left hepatic artery. Care should be taken here to identify any aberrant left hepatic artery anatomy, which is not uncommon. Careful attention should also be paid to the segment IV branch of the left hepatic artery. If this arises proximally off the left hepatic artery and appears to provide significant inflow to segment IV, this should be re-anastomosed to the right-sided grafts gastroduodenal artery remnant [14]. Control of the left hepatic duct and the left portal vein is similarly obtained. Portal venous branches to segment 4 should be ligated to fully expose the left portal vein. The liver parenchyma is divided with electrocautery or other hemostatic device approximately 1cm lateral to the falciform ligament and carried down to the level of the bile duct, at which point the parenchyma is sharply transected. Any small vessels or biliary radicles encountered along the way are oversewn as appropriate. The left hepatic vein, left hepatic artery, and left portal vein are then sharply divided. The left lateral segment graft can then be removed with its attached vascular and biliary system. The remainder of the right-sided graft can then be removed in the usual fashion.

The second variant involves creating two roughly equivalent hemi-livers (I-IV and V-VIII), either for two adult recipients or an adult and an older child. This is decidedly more complex due to the need to transect more hepatic parenchyma, higher chance of altering vascularization of each hemi-liver, and a less well-defined plane of transection (compared to the falciform ligament defining the left lateral segment). Initial dissection is similar to splitting the left lateral segment. The hepatic veins and the hepatoduodenal ligament are identified and individual structures dissected out. Care should be taken here to preserve the segment IV branches arising from the left hepatic artery. Identification of the line of parenchymal transection can be done by occluding the left portal vein and left hepatic artery, thereby stopping inflow to the left hemi-liver. A line of demarcation will appear and can be marked with electrocautery. The left hepatic duct is transected at the hilar plate, and parenchymal transection can proceed along the main portal fissure. Parenchymal division should stay just lateral to the middle hepatic vein so that this remains with the left lobe. Again, any small vessels or biliary radicles encountered along the way are oversewn. The right portal vein is transected just after its takeoff from the main portal vein, and the right hepatic artery is transected just after its take off from the common hepatic artery. The right hepatic vein is generally removed with a small patch of inferior vena cava to facilitate later anastomosis. The right hemi-liver is then removed, and the left-sided graft can be removed following standard procurement techniques.

Donor and Recipient Selection

Given the inherent risks of splitting a liver, and the potential to damage the scarce resource that a donor organ represents, careful attention must be paid both to what types of donors are chosen for this technique and which recipients are appropriate for split livers. In general, donor organs must be of relatively high quality to be considered appropriate for splitting. The loss of functional liver mass associated with splitting a liver means that both grafts obtained from splitting need to be of high quality to prevent primary non-function following transplantation. Since 2007, national match runs have identified a donor liver as being a candidate for splitting if the following criteria are met [15]:

• Donor less than 40 years old
• Donor transaminases less than three times normal limit
• Donor body-mass index less than 28
• Donor on no more than a single vasopressor dose

Beyond these criteria, an ideal donor should not have had a prolonged intensive care unit stay prior to donation. Obesity, hyper-/hypo-natremia, low platelet count, or a history of alcohol or drug abuse are relative contraindications to SLT [16]. Finally, intra-operative visualization of liver quality is critical, and any suspicions about quality should prompt liver biopsy. Mild abnormalities in the setting of an otherwise acceptable donor should probably not halt the decision to proceed with liver splitting.

Choosing the appropriate recipients for SLT follows the same general principles as selecting candidates for traditional whole liver transplantation. However, choosing an appropriately sized graft for each recipient is paramount. In general, the right extended graft (I, IV-VIII) obtained from a left lateral liver split has a volume of about 1000-1200cc, providing sufficient liver mass for a normal-sized adult [14, 17]. Additionally, this extended graft has a generous venous outflow and less susceptibility to venous congestion for patients in whom this is a concern. The left lateral segment (II, III) has a volume of about 250 cc and is appropriate for a pediatric recipient [17]. When SLT is done to produce two hemi-livers (I-IV, V-VIII), the left lobe (I-IV) will generally be around 400-600cc and can be generally transplanted into recipients of up to 65 kg, usually older children or small adults [14, 18]. The right lobe (V-VIII) has a volume of about 800-1000 cc and can be transplanted into recipients of up to 85 kg [14]. In general, most centers aim for a graft weight at least 1% of recipient body weight.

Potential Complications and Issues

One of the most feared complications following SLT is "small for size" syndrome. In this syndrome, the donor graft has inadequate liver mass to support the metabolic demands required by the patient following transplantation [19, 20]. As a result, the patient develops liver failure and potentially severe morbidity or mortality. While no single consensus definition has been settled on, it can broadly be characterized as prolonged cholestasis, coagulopathy, and ascites for more than seven days following partial graft liver transplantation. Of note, other complications such as vascular thrombosis, rejection, or sepsis must be ruled out first as any of these can mimic the clinical features of small for size syndrome. In general, it is seen when graft weight to recipient weight ratio is less than 0.8. One proposed definition requires two of the following to be present [19]:

- Hyperbilirubinemia (> 10 mg/dl)
- Coagulopathy (INR > 2)
- Moderate ascites
- Encephalopathy (grade 3 or 4)

It is worth noting that this syndrome can still develop even with a graft weight to recipient weight ratio that is more than 0.8, and in many series even the majority of patients with a ratio less than 0.8 do not develop small for size syndrome [20, 21]. In general, small for size syndrome is a rare occurrence in the pediatric population, occurring in <5% of all such recipients [22, 23].

As with traditional liver transplantation, a variety of complications occur following SLT. Specific complications occurring following pediatric SLT have not been extensively studied, but those studies that have been performed have identified several "major" types of complications: biliary, vascular, gastrointestinal, and re-transplantation. Of the "major" complications that can occur following pediatric SLT, biliary complications tend to happen most commonly, occurring in anywhere from 3-20% of such recipients [17, 24 - 26]. These consist mainly of biliary leak, often from the cut surface of the liver that occurs during splitting, although biliary strictures do occur as well. Vascular complications occur in less than 10% of all pediatric SLT recipients, and largely consists of hepatic artery thrombosis, although portal vein thrombosis occurs as well [17, 24 - 26]. Gastrointestinal complications (*i.e.* bowel perforation) are similarly rare, occurring in <5% of patients [24]. Finally, re-transplantation is necessary with some regularity, occurring in as many as 20% of all recipients [24 - 26].

Modern Outcomes

Fortunately, despite the poor outcomes reported early in the development of SLT, modern outcomes are excellent. Refinement in surgical technique and a better understanding of the types of donors and recipients appropriate for splitting have led to improved outcomes. A number of studies have examined patient and graft survival following SLT, and have consistently shown excellent results, with 5-year patient and graft survival generally exceeding 80% and 70% respectively [17, 24 - 29]. Several of these studies have directly compared pediatric recipients receiving a left lateral segment graft to those receiving whole deceased donor organs, and there has been no consistent difference in either survival or complication rate [24, 26 - 28]. This suggests that SLT is just as effective as whole organ deceased donor transplantation, and represents an excellent method for expanding the donor pool and improving access to liver transplantation.

LIVING DONOR LIVER TRANSPLANTATION

Introduction

Another technique used to expand access to liver transplantation is living donor liver transplantation (LDLT). Although initially attempted as early as 1998, the first successful LDLT was not performed until 2000 [30]. Soon after, the technique quickly gained acceptance and spread across the country. Since then, pediatric LDLT has been performed for virtually every indication for pediatric liver transplantation, including biliary atresia, metabolic disease, acute liver failure, neoplastic disease, and vascular disease [31 - 35] However, LDLT still represents a minority of all PLT in the United States. In 2014, only 52 pediatric recipients received a LDLT, little more than 10% of all pediatric liver transplants that year [36]. Interestingly, there are striking national differences in terms of the utilization of LDLT. In many Asian countries, for example, LDLT comprises a majority of liver transplantation, in part due to public mistrust of government-led deceased donor allocation systems and societal skepticism about the concept of brain death and cadaveric donation as a whole [37].

Although less commonly performed in the United States, pediatric LDLT represents an attractive technique to expand the potential donor pool and facilitate transplantation. LDLT offers a number of advantages compared to deceased donor liver transplantation. Generally, LDLT allows transplantation to happen on an elective basis when the recipient has had their medical, nutritional, and functional status optimized. This also helps avoid middle of the night or emergency operations. Additionally, less time is spent on the waiting list, preventing clinical worsening or even mortality in the time period leading up to transplantation. Despite these advantages, pediatric LDLT is not without its disadvantages. LDLT generally requires a dedicated living donor program and sufficient hepatobiliary expertise to assist with both the donor hepatectomy and transplantation into the recipient that not all programs are able to provide. Moreover, the living donor incurs the risks inherent to surgery and actual donation of the liver that unfortunately cannot be eliminated.

Donor Issues

One of the biggest obstacles for wider-spread adoption of pediatric LDLT in the United States is the fact that living donors derive no tangible benefit from donating, yet expose themselves to potential complications and even mortality by proceeding with donation. As with adult LDLT, care must be taken to make sure the donation process is undertaken with an appropriate understanding of the risks of donations. The possibility of death following hepatectomy should be discussed. In practice, this risk appears to be exceedingly small, occurring in <0.1% of all living donor hepatectomies [32, 38, 39]. Complications related to the donor hepatectomy occur in less than 20% of all donors, although much of this data comes from the adult literature [32, 38, 39]. Of these complications, the most common appear to be bile leak, intra-abdominal fluid collection, and wound infection. When evaluated using the Clavien classification system of complications, all but a very few of these complications are grade III or lower. Overall, the donor hepatectomy operation is relatively safe, although clearly there is still the potential for serious morbidity or mortality. All of this should be discussed with the potential donor.

To ensure an appropriate informed consent process takes place, it is important to have multiple discussions with the potential donor to ensure complete understanding of potential risks. Despite best efforts to fully inform the potential donor, in one study only 77% of living donors for pediatric liver transplantation felt "very well" or "well" informed about potential risks [32]. With pediatric LDLT, the donor is most often a parent. Rarely, a grandparent or older sibling will be the donor. In these cases, providing a liver for their child or close relative may be very gratifying, but care must be taken to guarantee the donation is in no way coerced. In one study, as many as 24% of living donors reported that they "may have" been coerced or pressured in some way into donating their organ, although no one reported being "forced" to do so [32]. Nevertheless, over 96% of those donors felt "no regret" with deciding to donate [32]. All of this should be kept in mind when discussing the donation process with a potential donor. Once a suitable and altruistic donor is identified for a child, the normal medical and psychiatric evaluation, described elsewhere, should proceed as normal.

Technical Issues

For pediatric LDLT, the donor operation is usually a left lateral segmentectomy (segments II and III). The operation proceeds similarly to the left lateral segment split described previously, with some differences noted below. The left hepatic vein is isolated, and attention is turned to the hepatoduodenal ligament. The left hepatic artery is dissected out as is the left portal vein. The left hepatic duct should be isolated as well, although this may not be possible prior to parenchymal transection. Parenchymal transection follows a line approximately 1cm lateral to the falciform ligament, and is carried out using some form of hemostatic device. A Pringle maneuver can be performed although this is not necessary. The left hepatic duct is sharply transected when encountered and the rest of the hepatic parenchyma divided. The left hepatic vein, left hepatic artery, and left hepatic vein are then divided sharply and the donor graft can be removed. This technique can be performed either open or laparoscopically as surgeon expertise permits. In very small children, the left lateral segment can be further reduced in size if necessary to keep the liver graft to recipient weight ratio less than 4%.

Potential Complications and Issues

One potential issue that is a particular problem in young infants undergoing liver transplantation is the "large for size" syndrome. As opposed to "small for size" syndrome, which occurs when liver graft to recipient weight ratio is less than 0.8%, the "large for size" syndrome occurs in general when the liver graft to recipient weight ratio exceeds 4%. This syndrome is characterized by poor graft perfusion and graft compression that leads to a higher incidence of vascular complications and hence poorer outcomes [40]. In very small children or young infants, when "large for size" syndrome is a possibility, special attention should be paid to the size of graft being obtained for the recipient. Some centers have used reduced size left lateral segment grafts or even monosegment grafts with similar outcomes to traditional left lateral segment transplantation.

Similar to traditional liver transplantation, a variety of complications can occur following pediatric LDLT. As with SLT, complications following LDLT can be divided into several "major" categories, and of these the vascular and biliary complications occur most commonly. Vascular complications occur in about 10-20% of all recipients, and tend to be evenly split between hepatic artery thrombosis and portal vein thrombosis [41 - 44]. Both can lead to graft loss and many centers routinely screen with duplex ultrasonography for some time following transplantation. Biliary complications, generally bile leak or biliary stricture, occur in 5-20% of patients [45, 46]. There does not appear to be a consistent relationship between reconstruction method (duct-to-duct or hepaticojejunostomy) for the biliary anastomosis and development of biliary complications [46]. Finally, re-transplantation is infrequent, and in one large study was only necessary in just over 6% of all pediatric LDLT recipients [47].

Modern Outcomes

Outcomes for pediatric LDLT are generally excellent, with 5-year patient and graft survival exceeding 80% and 70%, respectively [34, 48 - 50]. When compared to deceased donor liver transplantation, either whole liver or split graft, there have been no consistent differences in either patient or graft survival. The excellent long-term survival of pediatric LDLT in combination with its known advantages suggest LDLT should be continued to be pursued by the transplant community

SUMMARY

Pediatric liver transplantation is an effective therapy for end-stage liver disease and is associated with good long-term outcomes. Distinct from adult transplantation, pediatric liver transplantation is complicated by the small size of the children and the lack of size-matched deceased donor livers available for transplantation. Two main techniques have emerged to attempt to improve the situation: split liver transplantation and living donor liver transplantation. In general, both techniques allow the recipient smaller grafts, most often a left lateral segment. Split liver transplantation allows for two recipients to receive a liver transplant from a single donor organ, with no reduction in survival compared to whole organ transplantation. Living donor liver transplantation leverages a recipient's living donor to facilitate transplantation in an elective setting where recipient status can be optimized to the extent possible. Both techniques afford similar survival rates. Complications are common in both types of transplantation, with biliary and vascular complications generally occurring most frequently. Unfortunately, neither technique is commonly performed in the United States. Future efforts to expand the donor pool and minimize wait list mortality for pediatric liver transplant candidates should focus on expanding use of these proven techniques.

CONSENT FOR PUBLICATION

Not applicable.

CONFLICT OF INTEREST

The author declares no conflict of interest, financial or otherwise.

ACKNOWLEDGEMENTS

Declared none.

REFERENCES

[1] Devictor D, Tissieres P. Pediatric liver transplantation: where do we stand? Where we are going to? Expert Rev Gastroenterol Hepatol 2013; 7(7): 629-41.
[http://dx.doi.org/10.1586/17474124.2013.832486] [PMID: 24070154]

[2] Hackl C, Schlitt HJ, Melter M, Knoppke B, Loss M. Current developments in pediatric liver transplantation. World J Hepatol 2015; 7(11): 1509-20.
[http://dx.doi.org/10.4254/wjh.v7.i11.1509] [PMID: 26085910]

[3] Kamath BM, Olthoff KM. Liver transplantation in children: update 2010. Pediatr Clin North Am 2010; 57(2): 401-14.
[http://dx.doi.org/10.1016/j.pcl.2010.01.012] [PMID: 20371044]

[4] Spada M, Riva S, Maggiore G, Cintorino D, Gridelli B. Pediatric liver transplantation. World J Gastroenterol 2009; 15(6): 648-74.
[http://dx.doi.org/10.3748/wjg.15.648] [PMID: 19222089]

[5] Fouquet V, Alves A, Branchereau S, *et al.* Long-term outcome of pediatric liver transplantation for biliary atresia: a 10-year follow-up in a single center. Liver Transpl 2005; 11(2): 152-60.
[http://dx.doi.org/10.1002/lt.20358] [PMID: 15666395]

[6] UNOS/OPTN Data; https://optn.transplant.hrsa.gov/data accessed 8/21/17

[7] Massie AB, Chow EK, Wickliffe CE, *et al.* Early changes in liver distribution following implementation of Share 35. Am J Transplant 2015; 15(3): 659-67.
[http://dx.doi.org/10.1111/ajt.13099] [PMID: 25693474]

[8] Muller E, Kahn D, Mendelson M. Renal transplantation between HIV-positive donors and recipients. N Engl J Med 2010; 362(24): 2336-7.
[http://dx.doi.org/10.1056/NEJMc0900837] [PMID: 20554994]

[9] Fisher RA. Living donor liver transplantation: eliminating the wait for death in end-stage liver disease? Nat Rev Gastroenterol Hepatol 2017; 14(6): 373-82.
[http://dx.doi.org/10.1038/nrgastro.2017.2] [PMID: 28196987]

[10] Pichlmayr R, Ringe B, Gubernatis G, Hauss J, Bunzendahl H. Transplantation of a donor liver to 2 recipients (splitting transplantation)--a new method in the further development of segmental liver transplantation. Langenbecks Arch Chir 1988; 373(2): 127-30.
[http://dx.doi.org/10.1007/BF01262776] [PMID: 3287073]

[11] Bismuth H, Morino M, Castaing D, *et al.* Emergency orthotopic liver transplantation in two patients using one donor liver. Br J Surg 1989; 76(7): 722-4.
[http://dx.doi.org/10.1002/bjs.1800760723] [PMID: 2670054]

[12] Broelsch CE, Emond JC, Whitington PF, Thistlethwaite JR, Baker AL, Lichtor JL. Application of reduced-size liver transplants as split grafts, auxiliary orthotopic grafts, and living related segmental transplants. Ann Surg 1990; 212(3): 368-75.
[http://dx.doi.org/10.1097/00000658-199009000-00015] [PMID: 2396888]

[13] de Ville de Goyet J. Split liver transplantation in Europe-1988 to 1993. Transplantation 1995; 59(10): 1371-6.
[http://dx.doi.org/10.1097/00007890-199505270-00002] [PMID: 7770921]

[14] Renz JF, Yersiz H, Reichert PR, *et al.* Split-liver transplantation: a review. Am J Transplant 2003; 3(11): 1323-35.
[http://dx.doi.org/10.1046/j.1600-6135.2003.00254.x] [PMID: 14525591]

[15]   UNOS/OPTN. Split versus whole liver transplantation https://optn.transplant.hrsa.gov/media/1919/ethics_splitvwhole_livertx_20160815.pdf Accessed 8/25/17

[16]   Hashimoto K, Fujiki M, Quintini C, *et al.* Split liver transplantation in adults. World J Gastroenterol 2016; 22(33): 7500-6.
[http://dx.doi.org/10.3748/wjg.v22.i33.7500] [PMID: 27672272]

[17]   Yersiz H, Renz JF, Farmer DG, Hisatake GM, McDiarmid SV, Busuttil RW. One hundred *in situ* split-liver transplantations: a single-center experience. Ann Surg 2003; 238(4): 496-505.
[PMID: 14530721]

[18]   Humar A, Khwaja K, Sielaff TD, Lake JR, Payne WD. Technique of split-liver transplant for two adult recipients. Liver Transpl 2002; 8(8): 725-9.
[http://dx.doi.org/10.1053/jlts.2002.34680] [PMID: 12149768]

[19]   Goldaracena N, Echeverri J, Selzner M. Small-for-size syndrome in live donor liver transplantation-Pathways of injury and therapeutic strategies. Clin Transplant 2017; 31(2): e12885.
[http://dx.doi.org/10.1111/ctr.12885] [PMID: 27935645]

[20]   Chen PX, Yan LN, Wang WT. Outcome of patients undergoing right lobe living donor liver transplantation with small-for-size grafts. World J Gastroenterol 2014; 20(1): 282-9.
[http://dx.doi.org/10.3748/wjg.v20.i1.282] [PMID: 24415883]

[21]   Selzner M, Kashfi A, Cattral MS, *et al.* A graft to body weight ratio less than 0.8 does not exclude adult-to-adult right-lobe living donor liver transplantation. Liver Transpl 2009; 15(12): 1776-82.
[http://dx.doi.org/10.1002/lt.21955] [PMID: 19938139]

[22]   Vagefi PA, Parekh J, Ascher NL, Roberts JP, Freise CE. Outcomes with split liver transplantation in 106 recipients: the University of California, San Francisco, experience from 1993 to 2010. Arch Surg 2011; 146(9): 1052-9.
[http://dx.doi.org/10.1001/archsurg.2011.218] [PMID: 21931003]

[23]   Goldstein MJ, Salame E, Kapur S, *et al.* Analysis of failure in living donor liver transplantation: differential outcomes in children and adults. World J Surg 2003; 27(3): 356-64.
[http://dx.doi.org/10.1007/s00268-002-6598-8] [PMID: 12607066]

[24]   Doyle MB, Maynard E, Lin Y, *et al.* Outcomes with split liver transplantation are equivalent to those with whole organ transplantation. J Am Coll Surg 2013; 217(1): 102-12.
[http://dx.doi.org/10.1016/j.jamcollsurg.2013.03.003] [PMID: 23639200]

[25]   Moussaoui D, Toso C, Nowacka A, *et al.* Early complications after liver transplantation in children and adults: Are split grafts equal to each other and equal to whole livers? Pediatr Transplant 2017; 21(4): 1-9.
[http://dx.doi.org/10.1111/petr.12908] [PMID: 28261944]

[26]   Hong JC, Yersiz H, Farmer DG, *et al.* Longterm outcomes for whole and segmental liver grafts in adult and pediatric liver transplant recipients: a 10-year comparative analysis of 2,988 cases. J Am Coll Surg 2009; 208(5): 682-689, 689-691.
[http://dx.doi.org/10.1016/j.jamcollsurg.2009.01.023] [PMID: 19476815]

[27]   Broering DC, Mueller L, Ganschow R, *et al.* Is there still a need for living-related liver transplantation in children? Ann Surg 2001; 234(6): 713-21.
[http://dx.doi.org/10.1097/00000658-200112000-00002] [PMID: 11729377]

[28]   Cardillo M, De Fazio N, Pedotti P, *et al.* NITp Liver Transplantation Working Group. Split and whole liver transplantation outcomes: a comparative cohort study. Liver Transpl 2006; 12(3): 402-10.
[http://dx.doi.org/10.1002/lt.20720] [PMID: 16598843]

[29]   Cintorino D, Spada M, Gruttadauria S, *et al. In situ* split liver transplantation for adult and pediatric recipients: an answer to organ shortage. Transplant Proc 2006; 38(4): 1096-8.
[http://dx.doi.org/10.1016/j.transproceed.2006.02.146] [PMID: 16757275]

[30] Strong RW, Lynch SV, Ong TH, Matsunami H, Koido Y, Balderson GA. Successful liver transplantation from a living donor to her son. N Engl J Med 1990; 322(21): 1505-7.
[http://dx.doi.org/10.1056/NEJM199005243222106] [PMID: 2336076]

[31] Feier F, Schwartz IV, Benkert AR, *et al.* Living related *versus* deceased donor liver transplantation for maple syrup urine disease. Mol Genet Metab 2016; 117(3): 336-43.
[http://dx.doi.org/10.1016/j.ymgme.2016.01.005] [PMID: 26786177]

[32] Fukuda A, Sakamoto S, Shigeta T, *et al.* Clinical outcomes and evaluation of the quality of life of living donors for pediatric liver transplantation: a single-center analysis of 100 donors. Transplant Proc 2014; 46(5): 1371-6.
[http://dx.doi.org/10.1016/j.transproceed.2013.12.054] [PMID: 24836837]

[33] Hatanaka M, Nakazawa A, Nakano N, *et al.* Successful living donor liver transplantation for giant extensive venous malformation. Pediatr Transplant 2014; 18(5): E152-6.
[http://dx.doi.org/10.1111/petr.12280] [PMID: 24815871]

[34] Kasahara M, Sakamoto S, Sasaki K, *et al.* Living donor liver transplantation during the first 3 months of life. Liver Transpl 2017; 23(8): 1051-7.
[http://dx.doi.org/10.1002/lt.24743] [PMID: 28220684]

[35] Kim JS, Kim KM, Oh SH, *et al.* Liver transplantation for metabolic liver disease: experience at a living donor dominant liver transplantation center. Pediatr Gastroenterol Hepatol Nutr 2015; 18(1): 48-54.
[http://dx.doi.org/10.5223/pghn.2015.18.1.48] [PMID: 25866733]

[36] Kim WR, Lake JR, Smith JM, *et al.* Liver. Am J Transplant 2016; 16(S2) (Suppl. 2): 69-98.
[http://dx.doi.org/10.1111/ajt.13668] [PMID: 26755264]

[37] de Villa VH, Lo CM, Chen CL. Ethics and rationale of living-donor liver transplantation in Asia. Transplantation 2003; 75(3) (Suppl.): S2-5.
[http://dx.doi.org/10.1097/01.TP.0000046532.44975.57] [PMID: 12589129]

[38] Hashikura Y, Ichida T, Umeshita K, *et al.* Donor complications associated with living donor liver transplantation in Japan. Transplantation 2009; 88(1): 110-4.
[http://dx.doi.org/10.1097/TP.0b013e3181aaccb0] [PMID: 19584689]

[39] Iida T, Ogura Y, Oike F, *et al.* Surgery-related morbidity in living donors for liver transplantation. Transplantation 2010; 89(10): 1276-82.
[http://dx.doi.org/10.1097/TP.0b013e3181d66c55] [PMID: 20216482]

[40] Shehata MR, Yagi S, Okamura Y, *et al.* Pediatric liver transplantation using reduced and hyper-reduced left lateral segment grafts: a 10-year single-center experience. Am J Transplant 2012; 12(12): 3406-13.
[http://dx.doi.org/10.1111/j.1600-6143.2012.04268.x] [PMID: 22994696]

[41] Broniszczak D, Szymczak M, Kamiński A, *et al.* Vascular complications after pediatric liver transplantation from the living donors. Transplant Proc 2006; 38(5): 1456-8.
[http://dx.doi.org/10.1016/j.transproceed.2006.02.094] [PMID: 16797331]

[42] Moon JI, Jung GO, Choi GS, *et al.* Risk factors for portal vein complications after pediatric living donor liver transplantation with left-sided grafts. Transplant Proc 2010; 42(3): 871-5.
[http://dx.doi.org/10.1016/j.transproceed.2010.02.059] [PMID: 20430193]

[43] Seda-Neto J, Antunes da Fonseca E, Pugliese R, *et al.* Twenty years of experience in pediatric living donor liver transplantation: focus on hepatic artery reconstruction, complications, and outcomes. Transplantation 2016; 100(5): 1066-72.
[http://dx.doi.org/10.1097/TP.0000000000001135] [PMID: 27014791]

[44] Ueda M, Oike F, Kasahara M, *et al.* Portal vein complications in pediatric living donor liver transplantation using left-side grafts. Am J Transplant 2008; 8(10): 2097-105.
[http://dx.doi.org/10.1111/j.1600-6143.2008.02360.x] [PMID: 18727696]

[45] Byun J, Yi NJ, Lee JM, *et al.* Long term outcomes of pediatric liver transplantation according to age. J Korean Med Sci 2014; 29(3): 320-7.
[http://dx.doi.org/10.3346/jkms.2014.29.3.320] [PMID: 24616578]

[46] Miyagi S, Kawagishi N, Kashiwadate T, *et al.* Relationship between bile duct reconstruction and complications in living donor liver transplantation. Transplant Proc 2016; 48(4): 1166-9.
[http://dx.doi.org/10.1016/j.transproceed.2015.10.073] [PMID: 27320579]

[47] Ueda M, Oike F, Ogura Y, *et al.* Long-term outcomes of 600 living donor liver transplants for pediatric patients at a single center. Liver Transpl 2006; 12(9): 1326-36.
[http://dx.doi.org/10.1002/lt.20826] [PMID: 16773638]

[48] Kasahara M, Umeshita K, Inomata Y, Uemoto S. Long-term outcomes of pediatric living donor liver transplantation in Japan: an analysis of more than 2200 cases listed in the registry of the Japanese Liver Transplantation Society. Am J Transplant 2013; 13(7): 1830-9.
[http://dx.doi.org/10.1111/ajt.12276] [PMID: 23711238]

[49] Miura K, Sakamoto S, Shimata K, *et al.* The outcomes of pediatric liver retransplantation from a living donor: a 17-year single center experience. Surg Today. 2017. Published online April 22, 2017

[50] Yankol Y, Fernandez LA, Kanmaz T, *et al.* Results of pediatric living donor compared to deceased donor liver transplantation in the PELD/MELD era: Experience from two centers on two different continents. Pediatr Transplant 2016; 20(1): 72-82.
[http://dx.doi.org/10.1111/petr.12641] [PMID: 26861217]

CHAPTER 13

Islet Cell Donation

Jill Buss and **Amer Rajab**[*]

The Ohio State University, Columbus, OH, USA

Abstract: Islet cell transplantation has evolved as a viable alternative to solid organ pancreas transplantation. In this chapter, we review the important donor characteristics and techniques for successful islet cell procurement and transplantation.

Keywords: Islet Cell Donation, Pancreas Transplantation.

INTRODUCTION

Islet transplantation has emerged as an alternative to whole pancreas transplantation in the treatment of type 1 diabetes, particularly for patients who suffer from hypoglycemia unawareness. Islet transplantation allows for a minimally invasive surgery where isolated islets are infused into the liver of the recipient. Published data to date suggests that 2-3 infusions are optimal, however, in order to achieve insulin independence [1]. Therefore, multiple organ donors are required for effective treatment of each patient.

Pancreata used for islet isolation are generally selected from those that are not deemed acceptable for whole pancreas transplant. Therefore, the pool of potential donors is also limited. However, certain characteristics of donors that may exclude an organ from being used for whole pancreas transplantation may actually be preferable for use for islet transplantation. For example, donors with a high body mass index (BMI) are often rejected from use for whole pancreas transplant. But, studies have shown that a greater number of islets may be isolated from these donors, making them better suited as islet donors. In fact, donors with BMIs of $< 25 \text{ kg/m}^2$ usually result in islet isolation failures with islet doses that do not meet release criteria [2].

---

[*] **Corresponding author Amer Rajab:** The Ohio State University, Columbus, OH, USA; Tel: 614-293-6322; Fax: 614-293-4541; Email: amer.rajab@osumc.edu

Robert S.D. Higgins & Juan A. Sanchez (Eds.)

Donor Characteristics

Below are the general criteria used in screening donor pancreata for islet transplantation:

- Multi-organ donor
- Adequate in situ hypothermic perfusion infused through the distal aorta
- University of Wisconsin (UW) solution or Histidine-Tryptophan-Ketoglutarate (HTK) solution for perfusion and cold storage
- Maximum of 20 hours of cold ischemia time
- Donor age 15-75 years
- Mode of death – brain death secondary to craniocerebral trauma, spontaneous intracranial bleed, cerebrovascular accident, or primary brain tumor; non-hear--beating [donors after cardiac death (DCD)]
- Hospital stay < 96 hours
- Donor suitable for pancreas donation, but pancreas deemed unusable for whole organ pancreas transplantation by an experienced organ recovery or transplant surgeon using the general criteria (fibrosis, fatty, non-perforative duodenal trauma, pancreatic hematoma, non-reconstructable vascular anomaly)
- The following criteria for an otherwise acceptable organ donor would result in the exclusion of a pancreas for transplantation:
- Diabetes mellitus, type 1 or type 2
- Warm ischemia time > 30 minutes for heart-beating donors; warm ischemia time > 60 minutes for DCD donors
- Cold storage > 20 hours
- Prolonged hypotension causing pancreas dysfunction (increasing amylase and lipase levels) and/or biochemical abnormalities resulting in continuous rising of LFTs > 4 times normal
- Gross evidence of pancreatitis (possible consideration for islet but absolute exclusion for whole pancreas)
- Absolute contraindications for organ donation include:
- Active Hepatitis A, B, or C
- HIV or HTLV I or II positive
- Encephalitis
- Crutzfield-Jacob disease
- Rabies
- Tuberculosis
- Syphilis
- Septicemia
- Serious illness of unknown etiology
- Malignancy other than primary brain tumor
- Donor behavioral exclusion criteria for islet transplantation are as follows:

- Report of non-medical intravenous, intramuscular, or subcutaneous injection within 12 months preceding donation
- Hemophilia or related clotting disorder who have received human derived clotting factor concentrates
- Men/women who have engaged in prostitution in the last 5 years
- Sexual partners engaging in any of the above
- Persons exposed in the last 12 months to known or suspected HIV blood through accidental needle stick or contact with an open wound, non-intact skin or mucous membranes
- History of tattooing, ear/body piercing, or acupuncture within the last 12 months

Among organs that meet the above criteria and are determined to be acceptable for islet donation, many still are not usable following the isolation of the islet cells because the islet preparations do not meet release criteria for transplantation. Poor islet yield is the most common problem for failed islet isolations. Experience has shown that some donor characteristics may be associated with a greater likelihood for isolation success. Successful islet isolations for transplant have been associated with the following donor characteristics: age, BMI, cardiac arrest including hypotensive episodes and vasopressor dosage, blood glucose levels, and amylase levels [2].

Donor age has been shown to affect islet isolation success. Donors < 20 years of age have been shown to produce reduced islet yields [3, 4]. Some centers have shown the greatest islet yields from donors in the 45-50 year age range [2]. This success has been attributed to the collagen composition in the donor pancreas and the subsequent collagenase success in pancreas digestion. Conversely, however, the function of islets isolated from older donors has been shown to be reduced compared to younger donors. Therefore, the optimal donor age has been determined to be 20-45 years of age [5].

Donor BMI and body surface area (BSA) have also been shown to positively correlate with islet isolation success. A positive correlation has been shown to exist between donor weight and pancreas weight [6], and larger pancreata have been shown to contain more islets. According to islet donor scoring systems, donor BMIs between 25-30 kg/m^2 have been shown to be optimal, with some demonstrating success at BMIs up to 52 kg/m^2 [2].

Cold ischemia time (CIT) of the donor pancreas is also important to islet isolation success. Studies have shown that CIT of > 8 hours is associated with isolation failure [3, 4, 7]. Organ preservation methods may also play a role in isolation success. A multicenter study published in 2011 showed that the two-layer method (TLM) of pancreas preservation was preferable to preservation in the University of Wisconsin (UW) solution [8].

Donor Scoring

The North American Islet Donor Score (NAIDS) has been developed as a tool for identifying optimal pancreas donors for use in islet transplantation [9]. NAIDS was developed using data from 1,056 deceased donors across 11 centers in North America. In this scoring system, islet isolation success was defined as an islet yield after purification of > 400,000 islet equivalents. The NAIDS scoring system ranges from 0 to 100 as determined by univariate logistic regression analysis [9]. Two categories of donor variables emerged for correlation of donor scoring with islet isolation success. These categories include prediction of pancreas weight and pancreas quality. Prediction of pancreas weight utilizes donor data for age, gender, BSA, BMI, body weight and body height [9]. Donor characteristics used to predict pancreas quality include CIT, donor age, labs for pancreas, liver and kidney function, donor medical history, cause of death, duration of hospital stay, use of vasopressors and the team performing pancreas procurement [9]. There are three donor characteristics that most greatly influenced donor scoring. These included donor BSA, BMI, and the number of vasopressor types used.

Use of this scoring system allows for better predictability of successful islet isolations from donor pancreata. A higher NAIDS score is associated with a higher islet yield after isolation. Currently, there is no universal standard for what NAIDS score should be used as a cut off for donor eligibility. Each center performing islet transplantation may develop their own standards for determining acceptable donors based on NAIDS scoring.

Organ Procurement

Procurement of pancreata for islet transplantation is performed following the same standard protocol for procurement of a pancreas for whole organ transplantation. A standard sterile surgical technique is used to make a large midline incision in the abdomen with lateral extension at the level of the umbilicus. If the thoracic organs are also being procured, or if it is deemed necessary by the procuring surgeon, a sternotomy is performed. Then the right colon is mobilized to expose the distal aorta. The sub-diaphragmatic aorta is exposed and controlled. The spleen is mobilized with the tail of the pancreas. A Kocher maneuver is used to mobilize the duodenum and the head of the pancreas. The duodenum is transected using a gastrointestinal anastomosis stapler device just distal to the pylorus and distal to the ligament of Treitz. A dose of 30,000 units of heparin is administered, and the distal aorta is cannulated. The inferior mesenteric vein is cannulated as a route to the portal vein. The proximal sub-diaphragmatic aorta is cross-clamped and *in situ* flushing with chilled lactated

Ringer solution is started through the distal aorta and inferior mesenteric vein. After the *in situ* flush is completed, the pancreas is recovered. The pancreas is brought to the back table and flushed with chilled UW solution or HTK solution and cold stored at 4°C in the same solution. The organ is then transferred to the islet isolation laboratory. Labeling and packaging of the organ must meet United Network of Organ Sharing (UNOS) and Association of Organ Procurement Organizations (AOPO) standards. Typically, the pancreas is transported in cold UW solution (or HTK solution), protected by a triple sterile barrier. The outermost barrier must be a rigid container. The organ is then packed on ice in a biohazard cooler for transport to the isolation laboratory.

Upon receipt in the laboratory, the organ is logged into a product log sheet. The donor and recipient identifiers are verified. It must also be verified that the donor and recipient ABO blood types are compatible. A donor eligibility checklist label is completed by the islet transplant surgeon verifying that the donor screening, testing and medical history has been reviewed and meets eligibility requirements. CIT is documented and must be less than 20 hours to be used for clinical islet transplantation. The organ is washed in antibiotic and antimycotic wash solutions, rinsed in HBSS and weighed. An incision is made in the middle of the pancreas to expose the pancreatic duct. The duct is carefully cut and then cannulated on each side with an 18 gauge angiocatheter. The above steps may also be completed in the operating room immediately following organ procurement, prior to transporting the pancreas to the laboratory. Once the pancreatic duct is cannulated, islet isolation may begin.

Organ Preservation

Pancreata for islet transplantation are typically stored statically in either UW solution or HTK solution for up to 20 hours. Organs are stored cold to reduce cellular metabolism. The time from aortic cross clamp of the donor to the time of receipt of the organ in the isolation laboratory is referred to as the CIT. UW solution was developed in the 1980's for preservation of the liver, kidney and pancreas [10, 11]. It consists of a phosphate buffer system with a high potassium, low sodium electrolyte composition. Raffinose and lactobionic acid are included for osmotic membrane impermeability to prevent cellular edema [12]. HTK solution is a lower cost alternative to UW solution developed for kidney and liver preservation. It can also be used for pancreas preservation; however, studies have shown a reduction in graft survival following preservation of pancreata in HTK compared to UW solution [13]. An alternate organ preservation method called the two-layer method (TLM) for pancreas preservation has also been used and suggested to be potentially superior to using UW solution prior to islet isolation. The TLM was first introduced in 1988 and utilizes a perfluorochemical (PFC) solution in addition to UW solution. PFC is a hydrocarbon that can dissolve respiratory gases and release oxygen into surrounding tissue [14]. It is combined with an organ preservation solution (UW solution) that provides the necessary substrates for organ preservation. The lipophilic property and high density of PFC allows it to separate from the UW solution, forming two layers. The pancreas is surrounded by the UW solution and floats on oxygenated PFC [15].

Use of the TLM allows for oxygenation of the pancreas from the PFC solution during cold storage. It has been shown that an oxygen tension of about 60% of normal physiologic oxygen levels can be maintained using this method [16]. Use of this method has been shown to reduce ischemic reperfusion injury to the pancreas as well as reduce swelling [17] and improve the viability of the vascular endothelium [18] compared to storage in UW solution alone. Pancreas preservation using the TLM prior to islet isolation has been shown to increase islet yield, viability and *in vitro* function compared to storage in UW solution alone. It has also been suggested that the TLM may prevent trypsin activation, allowing for more effective collagenase delivery during pancreas digestion for islet isolation as well as protection of islets from collagenase digestion [19]. A 2015 meta-analysis of the TLM compared to the UW solution storage method prior to human islet isolation found that pancreas preservation using the TLM produced significantly higher islet yields compared to UW solution alone. However, there was no significant difference in islet viability or *in vitro* islet function [20]. Another meta-analysis published in 2011 showed that improvement of islet yield following use of the TLM was only evident when the TLM was used following UW storage or when there was a prolonged CIT (>20 hours). Benefits of the TLM for short-term storage were not clear [21].

CONCLUSION

Islet transplantation in the treatment of type 1 diabetes mellitus has made great advances in the past two decades. However, it is still a developing field. Improvements in islet yield and quality are vital to the continued success of the field of allogeneic islet transplantation due to the need for multiple donors and the current limited pool of organs. Further studies in pancreas preservation would assist in better islet isolation outcomes, and establishment of a universal scoring standard for islet donors would be helpful in optimizing islet products. Continued research will help to define the optimal criteria for islet donor selection as well as organ preservation and processing and bolster the success of islet transplants in the future.

CONSENT FOR PUBLICATION

Not applicable.

CONFLICT OF INTEREST

The author declares no conflict of interest, financial or otherwise.

ACKNOWLEDGEMENTS

Declared none.

REFERENCES

[1]   Shapiro AM, Lakey JR, Ryan EA, *et al.* Islet transplantation in seven patients with type 1 diabetes mellitus using a glucocorticoid-free immunosuppressive regimen. N Engl J Med 2000; 343(4): 230-8.
        [http://dx.doi.org/10.1056/NEJM200007273430401] [PMID: 10911004]

[2]   Berkova Z, Saudek F, Girman P, *et al.* Combining donor characteristics with immunohistological data improves the prediction of islet isolation success. J Diabetes Res 2016; Article ID 4214328: 8 pages.

[3]   Lakey JRT, Warnock GL, Rajotte RV, *et al.* Variables in organ donors that affect the recovery of human islets of Langerhans. Transplantation 1996; 61(7): 1047-53.
        [http://dx.doi.org/10.1097/00007890-199604150-00010] [PMID: 8623183]

[4]   Toso C, Oberholzer J, Ris F, *et al.* Factors affecting human islet of Langerhans isolation yields. Transplant Proc 2002; 34(3): 826-7.
        [http://dx.doi.org/10.1016/S0041-1345(01)02925-6] [PMID: 12034198]

[5]   Niclauss N, Bosco D, Morel P, *et al.* Influence of donor age on islet isolation and transplantation outcome. Transplantation 2016; 100(7): S848.
        [PMID: 21344706]

[6]   Kin T, Murdoch TB, Shapiro AM, Lakey JRT. Estimation of pancreas weight from donor variables. Cell Transplant 2006; 15(2): 181-5.
        [http://dx.doi.org/10.3727/000000006783982133] [PMID: 16719052]

[7]   Caballero-Corbalán J, Brandhorst H, Malm H, *et al.* Using HTK for prolonged pancreas preservation prior to human islet isolation. J Surg Res 2012; 175(1): 163-8.
        [http://dx.doi.org/10.1016/j.jss.2011.03.012] [PMID: 21550052]

[8]   Qin H, Matsumoto S, Klintmalm GB, De Vol EB. A meta-analysis for comparison of the two-layer and university of Wisconsin pancreas preservation methods in islet transplantation. Cell Transplant 2011; 20(7): 1127-37.
        [http://dx.doi.org/10.3727/096368910X544942] [PMID: 21092403]

[9]   Wang LJ, Kin T, O'Gorman D, *et al.* A multicenter study: North American islet donor score in donor pancreas selection for human islet isolation for transplantation. Cell Transplant 2016; 25(8): 1515-23.
        [http://dx.doi.org/10.3727/096368916X691141] [PMID: 26922947]

[10]   Wahlberg JA, Love R, Landegaard L, Southard JH, Belzer FO. 72-hour preservation of the canine pancreas. Transplantation 1987; 43(1): 5-8.
        [http://dx.doi.org/10.1097/00007890-198701000-00002] [PMID: 3541322]

[11]   Southard JH, van Gulik TM, Ametani MS, *et al.* Important components of the UW solution. Transplantation 1990; 49(2): 251-7.
        [http://dx.doi.org/10.1097/00007890-199002000-00004] [PMID: 1689516]

[12]   Petrowsky H, Clavien P-A. Principles of liver preservation.Transplantation of the liver. 3rd ed. Philadelphia, PA: Elsevier Saunders 2015; pp. 582-99.
        [http://dx.doi.org/10.1016/B978-1-4557-0268-8.00044-0]

[13]   Stewart ZA, Cameron AM, Singer AL, Dagher NN, Montgomery RA, Segev DL. Histidine-tryptophan-ketoglutarate (HTK) is associated with reduced graft survival in pancreas transplantation.

Am J Transplant 2009; 9(1): 217-21.
[http://dx.doi.org/10.1111/j.1600-6143.2008.02449.x] [PMID: 18986383]

[14]   Lowe KC, Davey MR, Power JB. Perfluorochemicals: their applications and benefits to cell culture. Trends Biotechnol 1998; 16(6): 272-7.
[http://dx.doi.org/10.1016/S0167-7799(98)01205-0] [PMID: 9652139]

[15]   Fujino Y. Two-layer cold storage method for pancreas and islet cell transplantation. World J Gastroenterol 2010; 16(26): 3235-8.
[http://dx.doi.org/10.3748/wjg.v16.i26.3235] [PMID: 20614478]

[16]   Matsumoto S, Kuroda Y, Hamano M, *et al.* Direct evidence of pancreatic tissue oxygenation during preservation by the two-layer method. Transplantation 1996; 62(11): 1667-70.
[http://dx.doi.org/10.1097/00007890-199612150-00023] [PMID: 8970625]

[17]   Tanioka Y, Kuroda Y, Kim Y, *et al.* The effect of ouabain (inhibitor of an ATP-dependent Na+/K+ pump) on the pancreas graft during preservation by the two-layer (University of Wisconsin solution/perfluorochemical) method following normothermic ischemia. Transplantation 1994; 57: 282-5.
[http://dx.doi.org/10.1097/00007890-199401001-00023] [PMID: 8310521]

[18]   Kuroda Y, Fujita H, Matsumoto S, *et al.* Protection of canine pancreatic microvascular endothelium against cold ischemic injury during preservation by the two-layer method. Transplantation 1997; 64(7): 948-53.
[http://dx.doi.org/10.1097/00007890-199710150-00002] [PMID: 9381539]

[19]   Matsumoto S, Rigley TH, Qualley SA, Kuroda Y, Reems JA, Stevens RB. Efficacy of the oxygen-charged static two-layer method for short-term pancreas preservation and islet isolation from nonhuman primate and human pancreata. Cell Transplant 2002; 11(8): 769-77.
[http://dx.doi.org/10.3727/000000002783985332] [PMID: 12588109]

[20]   Li X, Zhang J, Sang L, Chu Z, Dong M. Influence of the two-layer preservation method on human pancreatic islet isolation: a meta-analysis. Int J Artif Organs 2015; 38(3): 117-25.
[http://dx.doi.org/10.5301/ijao.5000391] [PMID: 25790972]

[21]   Qin H, Matsumoto S, Klintmalm GB, De Vol EB. A meta-analysis for comparison of the two-layer and university of Wisconsin pancreas preservation methods in islet transplantation. Cell Transplant 2011; 20(7): 1127-37.
[http://dx.doi.org/10.3727/096368910X544942] [PMID: 21092403]

CHAPTER 14

The Future of Organ Donation: *Ex Vivo* Preservation

Eliza Beal, Sylvester Black and **Bryan Whitson***

The Ohio State University, Columbus, OH, USA

Abstract: Extending the donor organ pool has been a long-standing goal of the transplant community given the inadequate supply of donor organs in comparison to the number of patients on the transplant waiting list. *ex vivo* preservation techniques are now evolving as a viable means to accomplish these goals. In this chapter, we review and explore the currently available techniques and potential for *ex vivo* preservation of solid organs.

Keywords: *Ex vivo* Liver Perfusion, *Ex vivo* Lung Perfusion, *Ex vivo* Preservation.

INTRODUCTION

There are shortages of both liver and lung grafts in the United States with demand far exceeding supply.

Ex Vivo Liver Perfusion

Due to a shortage of donor livers, there is increasing interest in *ex vivo* liver perfusion, which potentially provides the opportunity for both organ assessment and repair of marginal organs [1 - 3]. Cold static storage is easy to perform and is of low cost, however, there is ongoing damage and no opportunity for organ assessment or repair of marginal grafts. *Ex vivo* liver perfusion can be performed at hypothermic, subnormothermic, or normothermic temperatures. There are multiple commercial *ex vivo* liver perfusion platforms for normothermic *ex vivo* liver perfusion currently available including the OCS Liver PROTECT (Transmedics, Andover, MA), OrganOx Metra (OrganOx, Oxford, UK) and Liver Assist (Liver Assist, Groningen, the Netherlands).

---

* **Corresponding author Bryan Whitson:** The Ohio State University, Columbus, OH, USA; Tel: 614-293-8000; Email: bryan.whitson@osumc.edu

Robert S.D. Higgins & Juan A. Sanchez (Eds.)

Hypothermic Machine Perfusion

Hypothermic machine perfusion (HMP) is the standard in kidney transplantation, and has also been successfully applied to human liver transplantation [4 - 6, 8]. Hypothermic machine perfusion reduces the metabolic rate of the organ and leads to decreased production of inflammatory mediators [9]. Disadvantages of hypothermic machine perfusion secondary to the decreased metabolic rate included decreased ability to assess the organ during perfusion [1]. Its efficacy was first demonstrated in pre-clinical murine and porcine models [10 - 16]. These early murine studies demonstrated that in comparison to cold storage, HMP led to reduced production of reactive oxygen species, reduced caspase activity, improvements in alanine aminotransferase (ALT) and aspartate aminotransferase (AST) levels, reduced release of lactate dehydrogenase (LDH), maintained tissue adenine triphosphate (ATP), improved oxygen consumption, improved metabolic function as demonstrated by improved clearance of ammonia and production of urea, improved bile production, improved survival and suggested that HMP may reduce the early alloimmune response [10, 13, 14, 17, 18]. Early porcine studies demonstrated that grafts that underwent HMP with oxygenated perfusate at low portal venous pressures had reduced mitochondrial, nuclear and endothelial injury; and reduced Kupffer cell activation [19]. Furthermore, oxygenated HMP led to decreased aminotransferases, improved bile function, and reduced peribiliary ateriolonecrosis [16]. Additionally, efficacy of HMP has also been demonstrated using discarded human livers [20].

The efficacy of HMP has also been demonstrated in human studies. The first included 20 standard criteria grafts and showed that HMP provided protection as demonstrated by decreased AST, ALT and a shorter hospital stay than the historical control group [6]. The second included 8 donation after cardiac death (DCD) livers and demonstrated that recipient of HMP grafts had good early graft function and comparable AST, ALT, renal function and length of stay (LOS) as controls [7]. A third human study demonstrated in 31 extended criteria grafts that recipients of HMP grafts had lower ALT, creatinine, shorter LOS and significantly decreased incidence of biliary complications in comparison to controls [21].

Subnormothermic Perfusion

Subnormothermic machine perfusion (SNMP) is machine perfusion at 10-33 degrees Celsius, increasing the metabolic rate above HMP or cold storage and allowing for observation of graft function prior to transplantation. The use of SNMP has been demonstrated in both murine and porcine models. In comparison to cold storage these models, using both standard and steatotic livers, demonstrated decreased ALT, AST, and LDH and improved tissue ATP maintenance [22 - 24]. It was also demonstrated that tissue energy change (ATP/ADP ratio), oxidative stress and caspase activity were improved when livers were perfused at 20 degrees Celsius, but not when they were perfused at 4 degrees [23]. SNMP has also been used to deliver cryoprotectant to liver grafts prior to supercooling to -6 degrees Celsius – followed by successful rewarming and transplantation [25]. Pre-clinical comparisons of SNMP and HMP demonstrated that porcine livers undergoing SNMP after gradual rewarming to 20 degrees Celsius demonstrated decreased ALT release and improved bile production in comparison to HMP and controls [26]. In other comparisons of SNMP to cold storage, recipients of SNMP livers demonstrated improved bile duct preservation and function with decreased LDH in bile and the absence of biliary necrosis as well as improved endothelium maintenance on immunohistochemistry [27]. In a porcine standard criteria donor model with SNMP with a hemoglobin-based oxygen carrier, followed by transplantation, it was demonstrated that recipients of SNMP organs had decreased AST, ALT, improved bile production, and improved post-transplant survival [28]. In a porcine heart-beating donor graft model of SNMP, it was demonstrated that following transplantation recipients of SNMP grafts had reduced AST, alkaline phosphatase (ALP), hyaluronic acid and decreased sinusoidal cell apoptosis on immunohistochemistry in comparison to the cold storage group [29]. There are no clinical trials of SNMP, but Bruinsma *et al.* used discarded human grafts in a model of SNMP which demonstrated increasing oxygen uptake, increasing lactate clearance, increasing volume of bile production, improved ATP tissue maintenance, and preservation of hepatocyte morphology and sinusoidal endothelium [30]. The authors have also demonstrated the feasibility of using metabolomics to evaluate livers undergoing SNMP [31].

Normothermic Machine Perfusion

Normothermic machine perfusion (NMP) has many proposed advantages including decreased cold storage time, reduction in preservation injury, restoration of normal organ function under physiologic conditions, the ability to assess organ performance, and as a platform for organ repair, remodeling and modification [1, 32]. A multitude of pre-clinical murine and porcine studies have been done evaluating NMP.

A murine model of DCD organs underwent NMP at 20, 30 and 37 degrees Celsius and all had improved performance over cold storage organs with decreased AST, ALT, and improved post-transplantation survival (100% alive at 28 days *versus* 0%) in comparison to cold storage [33]. In another murine model of DCD livers that underwent NMP with or without prostaglandin E1, it was demonstrated that the prostaglandin E1 group had improved AST, ALT, decreased TNF-alpha, improved mitochondrial ATPase activity, decreased Bax and bcl-2 and reduced necrosis [34]. Some work has also been done in murine models to investigate opportunities for organ repair. Fatty livers from Zucker rats were isolated and underwent NMP with perfusate solution containing a combination of defatting agents. It was demonstrated that the intracellular lipid content of cells decreased by 50% over 3 hours [35]. In porcine studies, it has been demonstrated that NMP decreased ALT, AST, international normalized ratio (INR), hyaluronic acid levels, and bile duct necrosis, and improved oxygen consumption in comparison to cold storage [36, 37]. In a comparison of grafts undergoing 1 hour of cold storage and then 23 hours of NMP *versus* 24 hours of NMP, it was demonstrated that grafts that underwent a period of cold storage had significantly higher markers of cell damage including increased ALT and AST, sinusoidal dysfunction as demonstrated by increased hyaluronic acid, and increased beta-galactosidase indicating Kupffer cell injury [38]. An additional study comparing porcine livers that underwent NMP for 8 hours, underwent CS for 4 hours and then NMP for 4 hours and underwent CS for 4 hours and then were gradually rewarmed, demonstratimg that organs who underwent immediate NMP had lower liver transaminases, hyaluronic acid, beta-galactosidase, and higher bile production compared to other groups [39]. This suggests that periods of cold storage should be avoided prior to NMP. It has also been demonstrated in a porcine model that there were no differences between NMP and cold storage at short perfusion times (5 hours), but that at longer perfusion times (20 hours) there was improved survival in the NMP group. The authors also examined factors that distinguished NMP recipient survivors from non-survivors and demonstrated significant differences in bile output, base excess, ALT, AST, hyaluronic acid, portal venous pressure and portal venous resistance [40]. Furthermore, porcine studies of NMP have demonstrated superior hepatic artery perfusion on CT angiography in NMP livers [36]. Some work has been done on porcine models to demonstrate the use of NMP to repair or remodel organs. Goldaracena *et al.* recently published a proof of concept paper in which miravirsen was delivered during NMP to inhibit miR-122 function and lead to suppression of hepatitis C virus (HCV) replication. Improved uptake of miravirsen in NMP *versus* CS was demonstrated and miR-122 sequestration and target gene depression were seen in NMP but not in CS. Additionally the authors demonstrated *in vitro* that miravirsen led to the suppression of HCV replication in the cells with established infection and prevented infection in pretreated cells [41]. The same group demonstrated that the addition of the anti-inflammatory mediators alprostadil, n-acetylcysteine, carbon monoxide and sevoflurane led to reduced bilirubin, peak AST, IL-6, TNF-alpha and galactosidase in comparison to CS group [42]. Before formal human studies were conducted, discarded human organs were used to test NMP. It was demonstrated that DCD grafts undergoing NMP demonstrated bile production, decreasing lactate and preserved architecture after preservation [43]. It was determined that it might be possible to distinguish between grafts based on the production of bile – with the high bile output group putting out >30 grams over 6 hours and the low bile output group putting out <20 grams over 6 hours [44]. Furthermore, using discarded human livers, it was demonstrated that an organ could undergo NMP for up to 24 hours with continued bile production and reduction in lactate, although livers perfused for this duration demonstrated increased levels of perfusate urea [45]. Twelve discarded human livers underwent 6 hours of NMP and it was demonstrated that NMP results in activation of fibrinolysis, but not coagulation, and that markers of fibrinolysis correlate significantly with markers of ischemia-reperfusion injury suggesting that high d-dimer after the start of NMP is a predictor of poor liver graft function [46].

Several human studies have been performed using NMP. The first, by Ravikumar *et al.* in the UK, performed NMP with 20 standard criteria grafts using the OrganOx Metra platform and Gelofusine (Braun, Mumbai, India), a colloid solution. They demonstrated that median peak AST was significantly lower in the NMP group and that 30-day survival was similar between groups [47]. Bral *et al.* report their single-center North American experience using NMP including 10 donor liver grafts (4 DCD), 9 of which were transplanted. They demonstrated that all transplanted livers were functional and that serum levels of transaminases, bilirubin, INR and lactate were similar between groups and the primary outcome, 30-day graft survival, did not differ between groups [48]. Selzner *et al.* report on 10 human liver grafts perfused on the OrganOx Metra platform with Steen and 3 units of erythrocytes in comparison to a historical control group. There were no differences in post-op graft function, intensive care unit (ICU) stay, hospital LOS. There were significant differences in complications (7 in CS group *vs.* 1 in NMP group) and NMP recipients had lower AST and ALT on post-op days 1-3. The authors conclude that Steen is easier to use in the United States where it is already FDA approved, *versus* Gelofusine, which was used by Ravikumar *et al.,* but is not approved for use in the United States [49]. The Liver Assist platform (Liver Assist, Groningen, the Netherlands) has also been used for NMP in two recently reported cases in which extended criteria grafts were preserved for prolonged periods of time [50, 51]. The safety and feasibility of using normothermic *ex vivo* liver perfusion (NMP) to repair marginal organs has been recently demonstrated, with the successful transplantation of five discarded livers following NMP in the UK. Furthermore, they demonstrated the utility of graft assessment during *ex vivo* liver perfusion, using both objective (perfusate/lactate, bile production, arterial/portal venous flow) and subjective (homogeneity of perfusion, parenchymal texture) criteria to assess organ viability [52]. But until very recently, no strict criteria for defining transplantable and non-transplantable liver grafts had been set forth. Mergental *et al.* define the following criteria for transplantation for livers undergoing NMP: 1. Perfuase lactate <2.5 mmol/L OR evidence of bile production by 2 hours of perfusion, 2. Perfusate pH > 7.30, 3. Arterial flow >150 mL/minute AND portal flow > 500 mL/minute, and 3. Homogenous perfusion with soft graft parenchyma [52]. The definition of which organs are considered transplantable will likely evolve over time – successful resuscitation with NMP of an organ that underwent 109 minutes of warm ischemia and 7 hours of cold storage and another with 160 minutes of warm ischemia and 6 hours of cold storage have also recently been reported [50, 53]. NMP may also allow increased use of steatotic livers by reducing risk of primary nonfunction and early graft dysfunction through mitigation of preservation injury incurred during cold storage and evaluation of organ quality [1]. Novel strategies for monitoring liver grafts on *ex vivo* liver perfusion circuits that have been proposed in the literature include the use of electron paramagnetic resonance (EPR) spectroscopy to detect reactive oxygen species production or the use of dynamic contrast-enhanced ultrasound to measure blood flow in micro- and macro-circulation [54, 55].

Future Directions in *Ex Vivo* Liver Perfusion

There are multiple ongoing phase I-III clinical trials of NMP and HMP and a selection of these are summarized in Table. **14.1**. Areas for further research in the arena of normothermic *ex vivo* liver perfusion include elucidation of cellular mechanisms of injury mitigation, investigation of methods of graft repair, determination of evidence based protocols for perfusion, evidence based criteria for determining viability/transplantability and determination of ideal perfusate solutions [1].

Table 14.1. Ongoing Clinical Trials in Normothermic and Hypothermic Machine Perfusion of the Liver.

Ongoing Clinical Trials in Normothermic and Hypothermic Machine Perfusion of the Liver			
Title	**Institution**	**Design / Status / Device**	**Outcomes**
A *Phase I* Pilot Study to Assess Safety and Feasibility of Normothermic Machine Preservation In Human Liver Transplantation (NCT02515708)	The Cleveland Clinic, Cleveland, OH	32 Livers, acceptable quality for transplantation, 4-18 hours NMP, 6 month post-transplantation follow-up, compared to 128 matched (age, MELD, preservation time) historical controls, recruiting Device: Normothermic Liver Perfusion Device	Primary outcome: EAD (bilirubin>= 10, INR>=1.6, AST > 2000 U/L), Secondary: PNF, graft survival, peak LFTs in first 7 days, intraoperative flow measurement, post-reperfusion syndrome, surgical outcomes, kidney failure, histology of liver parenchyma, biliary complication rate, hospital and ICU LOS, rejection rate, opportunistic viral infection rate, patient survival, histology of bile duct

(Table 14.1) cont.....

Ongoing Clinical Trials in Normothermic and Hypothermic Machine Perfusion of the Liver			
Title	**Institution**	**Design / Status / Device**	**Outcomes**
VITTAL: An Open Label, Non-randomised, Prospective, Single Arm, 2-part Trial, Using Normothermic Machine Liver Perfusion NMLP to Test Viability and Transplantation of Marginal Livers (NCT02740608)	University of Birmingham	Study population is extended criteria grafts rejected for transplantation from all UK centers and then found to be functioning during perfusion and transplanted into medium-to-low risk liver transplant recipients, recruiting, Device: OrganOx metra (Organox, Oxford, UK)	Primary outcome: patient survival, use of NMP to identify the proportion of transplantable liver grafts from currently rejected organ donor pool, Secondary: liver graft function (LFTs, 90-day graft survival, 12 month patient and graft survival), morbidity associated with receipt of extended criteria graft (adverse event rate and severity, requirement of renal replacement therapy, incidence of biliary complications, vascular complications, biopsy-proven acute rejection, reoperation rate, length of ICU stay, LOS, physiologic response to reperfusion of the graft
Assessing the Safety and Efficacy of a Portable *Ex Vivo* Oxygenated, Normothermic Liver Perfusion System (OrganOx Metra™) Prior to Liver Transplantation (Phase I and II) (NCT03089840)	University of Alberta	Estimated enrollment 50, donor organ placed in OrganOx metra device at donor institution and then transported, perfused for ≥ 4 hours, transplanted, patient managed according to standard protocols, compared to 100 historic matched controls, Device: OrganOx metra	Primary outcome: graft survival rate, Secondary: patient survival rate, EAD, peak AST, daily lactate, perfusate AST, perfusate ALT, perfusate bilirubin
A Double Blinded Randomized Study on the Effects of Hypothermic Oxygenated Perfusion (HOPE) on Human Liver Grafts Before Transplantation (Phase II) (NCT01317342)	University of Zurich	Estimated enrollment: 70, two-arm, one hour hypothermic perfusion *versus* control group, IGL solution as perfusate, followed for one year after transplantation, Device: Hypothermic Oxygenated Perfusion	Primary outcome: Postoperative peak ALT, postoperative outcome (Dindo/Clavien classification), LOS, length of ICU stay, inflammatory response and reperfusion injury, patient and graft survival, outcome in terms of extended criteria grafts

(Table 14.1) cont.....

Ongoing Clinical Trials in Normothermic and Hypothermic Machine Perfusion of the Liver			
Title	**Institution**	**Design / Status / Device**	**Outcomes**
A Multicenter Randomized Controlled Trial to Compare the Efficacy of End-ischemic Dual Hypothermic Oxygenated Perfusion With Standard Static Cold Storage of Liver Grafts Donated After Circulatory Death in Preventing Biliary Complications (Phase 3)	Erasmus Medical Center, Leiden University Medical Center	Estimated Enrollment: 156, Adult patients (≥18 yrs old) undergoing a liver transplantation with a liver graft procured from a controlled DCD donor (Maastricht category III) with a body weight ≥40 kg. In the intervention group liver grafts will be subjected to two hours of hypothermic, oxygenated perfusion at the end of SCS and before implantation. In the control group donor liver grafts will be preserved in accordance to standard practice by SCS only. Device: Liver Assist, Drug: Glutathione	Primary outcome: Incidence of symptomatic NAS, Secondary outcome: asymptomatic NAS, severity of NAS, location of NAS, graft survival, patient survival, primary nonfunction, initial poor function, blood pressure, heart rate, vasopressor dosage, LOS, postoperative complications, renal function, flow, pressure, resistance, new onset diabetes after transplantation, costs of treatment, health related quality of life, perfusate laboratory values and genetics
Hypothermic Oxygenated Machine Perfusion (HOPE) for Orthotopic Liver Transplantation of Human Liver Allografts From Extended Criteria Donors (ECD) in Donation After Brain Death (DBD); a Prospective Randomized Controlled Trial (HOPE ECD-DBD)	University Hospital Aachen	Experimental: HOPE for 1 hour *via* portal vein in a recirculating and pressure controlled system, 0.1 ml/gram liver/minute, perfusion volume 3-4 L, Belzer (UW) machine perfusion solution, temperature 4-6 degrees Celsius, perfusate oxygenation 60-80 kPa, Control: conventional cold storage at 4-6 degrees celsius, Device: Hypothermic Oyxgenated Perfusion (HOPE)	Primary outcome: Early graft dysfunction, Secondary: postoperative complications, cumulative postoperative complications, duration of ICU stay, LOS, one-year recipient and graft survival, ischemia-reperfusion injury and inflammatory response
A Single Centre Study of the Feasibility and Safety of Using *Ex vivo* Normothermic Machine Perfusion With the Organox Metra™ Device to Store Human Livers for	University of Toronto	Estimated Enrollment: 40, Examining feasibility of using OrganOx metra device to transport and store donor livers under normothermic conditions prior to transplantation. Will follow participants for	Primary outcome: rates of primary graft non-function, re-transplantation and recipient death; Secondary: rates of device failure resulting in organ discard, recruitment rates to the study, ischemia-reperfusion injury associated with organ storage, function of liver grafts stored with OrganOx metra device measured by bilirubin, alkaline phosphatase,

(Table 14.1) cont.....

Ongoing Clinical Trials in Normothermic and Hypothermic Machine Perfusion of the Liver			
Title	**Institution**	**Design / Status / Device**	**Outcomes**
Transplantation (Phase 1) (NCT02478151)	University of Toronto	3 months following transplantation.	AST, INR, the ability of perfusion parameters to predict clinical outcomes following transplantation including flow, pressure, blood gas and bile production

Ex Vivo Lung Perfusion

There is currently also a shortage of lung donors. Standard lung criteria for donation including donor age less than 55 years old, ABO compatible, approximate size match, clear chest x-ray, PaO_2/FiO_2 more than 300 on 5 mmHg of Positive End Expiratory Pressure (PEEP), tobacco history less than 20 pack-years, clear bronchoscopy and no primary pulmonary disease. Lungs that do not meet these criteria have been shown to be at higher risk of primary graft dysfunction, which is a common complication of lung transplantation including acute pulmonary edema associated with bilateral pulmonary infiltrates and hypoxemia in the first three post-operative days [56]. *Ex vivo* lung perfusion (EVLP) is one potential method of repairing organs that may fall outside these standard criteria in an effort to reduce the risk of primary graft dysfunction. *Ex vivo* lung perfusion also allows us to develop metrics to assess organ function, approaches to mitigate acute organ injury and recondition organs and modify or protect organs to enhance resistance to injury. It has been demonstrated that the use of EVLP could lead to a significant increase in available donors [57]. In an early prospective, nonrandomized clinical trial high-risk donor lungs (pulmonary edema, PaO_2/FiO_2 ratio less than 300) underwent four hours of EVLP. Lungs from 23 donors met criteria and in 20 lungs physiologic function remained stable and they were transplanted. These were compared to 116 control lungs transplanted during the same period. EVLP lungs demonstrated reduced incidence of primary graft dysfunction 72 hours after transplantation (15% *vs.* 30%, p=0.11) and no significant differences were observed in 30-day mortality, bronchial compli-cations, duration of mechanical ventilation and ICU and hospital length of stay. The authors concluded that high-risk donor lungs that undergo EVLP and are physiologically stable have similar outcomes to conventionally selected lungs [58].

ANIMAL MODELS

Porcine Models

Porcine models have been used to demonstrate the efficacy of EVLP with an acellular perfusate with or without additives in preserving and monitoring DCD lungs, sepsis-injured lungs and those damaged by gastric acid aspiration [59 - 63]. Targeted drug therapy with an adenosine A2B receptor agonist, ATL802, with EVLP, were shown to allow for successful transplantation of severely injured DCT lungs exposed to 2 hours of warm ischemia [60]. Porcine large animal survival models have been used to investigate potential to repair donor organs. The benefits of *ex vivo* adenoviral human interleukin-10 (Adhil-10) gene delivery to prevent primary graft dysfunction were explored and demonstrated that immediate post-transplant lung function was improved in the EVLP and Adhil-10 groups and histologic inflammation scores were lower [61]. Prevention of primary graft dysfunction using multipotent adult progenitor cells (MAPC) has also been explored; it was demonstrated that delivery of MAPC in the airways of porcine lungs led to a reduction in pro-inflammatory cytokines and neutrophils in bronchoalveolar lavage specimens [64]. Ability of lung lavage and surfactant administration to mitigate gastric acid aspiration-induced donor lung injury was also investigated using a large animal survival model. Gastric acid aspiration was induced in pigs and lungs were procured. The lavage and surfactant group demonstrated reduced inflammatory mediators, reduced hydrolysis of phosphatidylcholine and improved post-transplant lung function [62]. In a lipopolysaccharide induced porcine model of lung injury it was demonstrated that 4 hours of EVLP with STEEN Solution (XVIVO Perfusion Inc., Englewood, CO) successfully rehabilitated lungs [63]. Porcine models have also been used to explore the effects of steroids on warm ischemic injury – demonstrating that warm ischemic injury in donation after cardiac death donation can be mitigated by using steroids when given prior to warm ischemia and during EVLP [65]. Furthermore, it has been demonstrated using porcine models that lungs donated after circulatory death can be transplanted as many as 6 hours after EVLP has been completed when they undergo cold preservation. This could allow them to be transported to more distant recipients.

Rodent Models

Reproducible models for *ex vivo* lung perfusion in the rat have been published and used to explore various elements of *ex vivo* lung perfusion [66]. For example, using a rat model of EVLP, various perfusate oxygen levels were compared (6%, 40%, 60%, 100%) and it was noted that lungs perfused with 40% oxygen had the lowest glucose consumption, exhibited less inflammation than those perfused with

6% or 100%, had reduced oxidative damage in comparison to those perfused with 100% and had the best post-transplant outcomes [67]. A rat model of *ex vivo* perfusion of heart-lung blocks with use of a leukocyte filter demonstrated that removal of circulating leukocytes from donor lungs resulted in decreased caspase-1 induced cell death and improved quality of donor grafts [68]. However, the addition of a leukocyte filter was not found to be beneficial in a porcine EVLP model [69]. Pharmacologic reconditioning with EVLP has been explored extensively in murine models [70]. The innate immune inhibitor pyrrolidine dithiocarbamate delivery during EVLP was shown to improve the quality of damaged rat DCD lungs [70]. Various other molecules have been used in an effort to recondition lungs during EVLP including inhibitors peroxynitrite and ADP-ribose polymerase [71].

Human Observational Studies

A multi-center study involving all five UK adult lung transplant centers evaluated the clinical and cost effectiveness of EVLP in increasing UK lung transplant activity in patients aged 18 years and older. The primary outcome of this study was survival during the first 12 months after transplantation and the secondary outcomes were patient-centered outcomes and health-care costs. Only one third of donor lungs subjected to EVLP were eventually transplanted. Twelve month survival was lower in the EVLP group than in the standard group. There were also increased rates of primary graft dysfunction, high extracorporeal membrane oxygenation (ECMO) requirement and differences in lung injury in EVLP organs [72]. It has also been demonstrated that EVLP can be used to extend graft preservation time beyond 12 hours without negatively impacting transplantation outcomes [73].

Single center results comparing outcomes of recipients of EVLP and non-EVLP lungs have also been reported. In a Swedish study, 32 pairs of donor lungs which had been initially rejected underwent EVLP and 22 double lung and 5 single lungs were transplanted. These were compared to 145 patients who received conventional donor lungs during the same time period. There were no significant differences in median time to extubation, median intensive care unit stay, cumulative survival or freedom from retransplantation or chronic rejection [74]. In a German study, 322 consecutive lung transplants performed between January 2007 and December 2014 were divided into two groups based on the organ storage strategy employed (n=308 conventional cold storage, n=14 organ care system) and outcomes were compared. Those patients who received lungs which had been preserved with the organ care system had significantly improved postoperative FEV1 at 3 and 6 months and there were no significant differences in cumulative survival or freedom from bronchiolitis obliterans syndrome between the two groups.

Discarded Lungs

EVLP was performed on four human lungs and two which had acceptable lung function parameters underwent immunologic investigation which demonstrated that TNF-alpha, IL-6 and IL-8 were decreased in each stage of washing perfusate and that intra-capillary pools of pro-inflammatory cytokines were determined to contribute to the lung injury during prolonged lung perfusion, raising the possibility that EVLP donor lungs are less immunogenic than standard lungs [75]. Donor lungs are often rejected due to concern for infection. *Ex vivo* lung perfusion with high-dose antibiotics has been proposed as one potential treatment option and its use has been demonstrated to result in quantitative reductions in bacterial counts in bronchoalveolar lavage, reduced perfusate endotoxin levels, improved pulmonary oxygenation and compliance, and reduced pulmonary vascular resistance [76].

Biomarkers

In comparison to the liver, the quality of donor lungs is difficult to measure. This has spurred the search for biomarkers that could aid in donor lung assessment and/or allow continuous monitoring of lungs undergoing EVLP. In a study of 100 sequential EVLP patients including 79 lungs which were transplanted, it was demonstrated that levels of M30 and HMGB-1 in EVLP perfusate correlate with primary graft dysfunction after lung transplantation [77]. Measurement of exhaled carbon monoxide has been shown to be a potential biomarker of ischemia reperfusion injury during EVLP, as levels correlate with length of cold ischemia time [78]. In an effort to evaluate which biomarkers were efficacious in determining the difference between in-hospital survival and non-survival, longitudinal samples of perfusate, bronchoalveolar lavage and tissue from 42 human donor lungs undergoing EVLP were analyzed. Interleukin-1β ad tumor necrosis factor-α were the most effective. Interleukin-1β was proposed as a potential target for blockade [79]. Other methods of evaluating lung quality during EVLP have been proposed including the use of real-time computed tomography (CT) [80].

Published Trials

It has been demonstrated in clinical trials that EVLP can be used safely for standard donor lungs [58, 81]. The first clinical trial was published by the Toronto group in 2011 in the New England Journal of Medicine. This was a prospective, nonrandomized clinical trial in which lungs which were determined to be high risk for transplantation were subjected to 4 hours of EVLP. Lungs with acceptable function were then transplanted. The primary end point of this study was primary graft dysfunction 72 hours after transplantation and secondary endpoints included 30-day mortality, bronchial complications, duration of mechanical ventilation, and length of stay in the ICU and hospital. There were 136 lung transplantations performed during the study period, lungs from 23 donors met criteria for EVLP and 20 of these were later transplanted and compared to the other 116 lungs transplanted during this time period. There was no significant difference in primary graft dysfunction in the EVLP and control groups and there were also no significant differences between any of the secondary endpoints [58]. The Toronto group later published their results after 50 consecutive transplants after *ex vivo* lung perfusion and noted no difference in 30-day mortality or 1-year survival [82]. Functional outcomes were examined after 63 patients underwent transplantation with EVLP treated grafts – 1, 3, and 5-year survival, freedom from chronic allograft dysfunction, highest FEV1, and number of acute rejection episodes did not differ between groups. Additionally, both groups reported improvement in their quality of life and there was no difference between groups in improvement in quality of life [83]. A prospective randomized trial at the University of Vienna included 80 recipient/donor pairs – 41 control and 39 EVLP. Four lungs in the EVLP group were not transplantable. Total cold ischemic time was longer in the EVLP group. The EVLP group experienced lower incidence of primary graft dysfunction and decreased need for post-operative prolonged ECMO. Other short-term outcomes including intubation days, ICU length of stay, and hospital length of stay were not different between groups. There was no difference in 30-day survival between groups. The authors conclude that EVLP can be safely used in standard donor lungs with good outcomes and that EVLP can safely extend preservation time [81]. Using the Toronto method, a group from the University of Turin, reported on the outcomes of 28 standard and 8 EVLP lungs and determined that there were no significant differences in primary graft dysfunction immediately after lung transplantation or at 72 hours and no difference in post-transplant extracorporeal membrane oxygenation rates [84]. Similarly, a French group reported on 31 donor lungs transplanted after EVLP and 81 standard double-lung transplants. They demonstrated no difference in median time to extubation, ICU stay, hospital stay, 30-day mortality, or 1-year survival [85]. The Toronto group also reported their experience with donation after cardiac death lungs after undergoing *ex vivo* lung perfusion. Cases which underwent EVLP had shorter hospital stays and a trend towards shorter length of mechanical ventilation [86].

Ongoing Trials

There are a multitude of ongoing clinical trials examining the use of *ex vivo* lung perfusion including:

- the HELP trial sponsored by Vitrolife in Toronto and using extended criteria grafts;
- the NOVEL trial sponsored by XVIVO taking place in the United States and using extended criteria grafts and the XPS Flexible Comprehensive EVLP platform (Fig. **14.1**);
- the INSPIRE trial sponsored by Transmedics taking place in Europe and the United States and using standard grafts and portable technology;
- the EXPAND trial sponsored by Transmedics taking place in Europe and the United States using extended criteria grafts and portable technology;
- the DEVELOP trial sponsored by Vivoline taking place in the United Kingdom using extended criteria grafts, the Vienna trial sponsored by XVIVO and taking place in Vienna using standard grafts;
- the Perfusix trial taking place in the United States using extended criteria grafts [87].

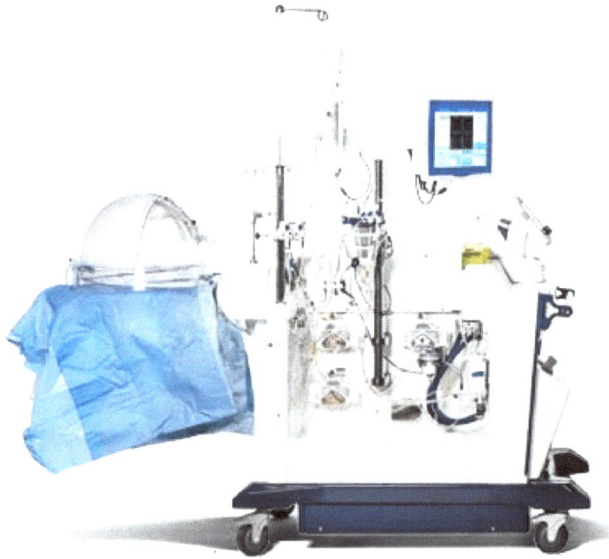

Fig. (14.1). The XVIVO Perfusion XPS Flexible Comprehensive EVLP Platform. Used with permission. Medical Illustrations© 2018 Tim Phelps, MS, FAMI, Johns Hopkins University.

FUTURE DIRECTIONS

Beyond expanding the donor pool for lung transplantation, other uses of *ex vivo* lung perfusion have also been proposed. One that is particularly intriguing is the use of *ex vivo* lung perfusion to preserve lungs for auto-transplantation during *ex vivo* resection or ablation of oligometastatic disease [88, 89]. Furthermore, *in vivo* lung perfusion with high dose chemotherapy to treat pulmonary metastatic disease has also been proposed [90].

CONCLUSION

Ex vivo liver and lung perfusion have both been demonstrated to be safe and effective methods of preserving organs prior to transplantation.

CONSENT FOR PUBLICATION

Not applicable.

CONFLICT OF INTEREST

The author declares no conflict of interest, financial or otherwise.

ACKNOWLEDGEMENTS

Declared none.

REFERENCES

[1]   Barbas AS, Knechtle SJ. Expanding the donor pool with normothermic *ex vivo* liver perfusion: the future is now. Am J Transplant 2016; 16(11): 3075-6.
[http://dx.doi.org/10.1111/ajt.13959] [PMID: 27402131]

[2]   OPTN OPaTN. National Data, Transplants by Donor Type, U.S. Transplants Performed January 1, 1988 - December 31, 2016, For Organ = Liver 2017. Available from: https://optn.transplant.hrsa.gov/data/view-data-reports/national-data/#

[3]   OPTN OPaTN. National Data. Organ by Status. Current U.S. Waiting List For Type = Registrations Based on OPTN data as of February 7 2017 2017. Available from: https://optn.transplant.hrsa.gov/data/view-data-reports/national-data/#

[4]   Moers C, Smits JM, Maathuis MH, *et al.* Machine perfusion or cold storage in deceased-donor kidney transplantation. N Engl J Med 2009; 360(1): 7-19.
[http://dx.doi.org/10.1056/NEJMoa0802289] [PMID: 19118301]

[5]   Jochmans I, Moers C, Smits JM, *et al.* Machine perfusion *versus* cold storage for the preservation of kidneys donated after cardiac death: a multicenter, randomized, controlled trial. Ann Surg 2010; 252(5): 756-64.
[http://dx.doi.org/10.1097/SLA.0b013e3181ffc256] [PMID: 21037431]

[6]   Guarrera JV, Henry SD, Samstein B, *et al.* Hypothermic machine preservation in human liver transplantation: the first clinical series. Am J Transplant 2010; 10(2): 372-81.
[http://dx.doi.org/10.1111/j.1600-6143.2009.02932.x] [PMID: 19958323]

[7]   Dutkowski P, Schlegel A, de Oliveira M, Müllhaupt B, Neff F, Clavien PA. HOPE for human liver grafts obtained from donors after cardiac death. J Hepatol 2014; 60(4): 765-72.
[http://dx.doi.org/10.1016/j.jhep.2013.11.023] [PMID: 24295869]

[8]   O'Callaghan JM, Morgan RD, Knight SR, Morris PJ. Systematic review and meta-analysis of hypothermic machine perfusion *versus* static cold storage of kidney allografts on transplant outcomes. Br J Surg 2013; 100(8): 991-1001.
[http://dx.doi.org/10.1002/bjs.9169] [PMID: 23754643]

[9]   Barbas AS, Goldaracena N, Dib MJ, Selzner M. *Ex vivo* liver perfusion for organ preservation: Recent advances in the field. Transplant Rev (Orlando) 2016; 30(3): 154-60.
[http://dx.doi.org/10.1016/j.trre.2016.03.002] [PMID: 27158081]

[10]   Dutkowski P, Furrer K, Tian Y, Graf R, Clavien PA. Novel short-term hypothermic oxygenated perfusion (HOPE) system prevents injury in rat liver graft from non-heart beating donor. Ann Surg 2006; 244(6): 968-76.
[http://dx.doi.org/10.1097/01.sla.0000247056.85590.6b] [PMID: 17122622]

[11]   Fondevila C, Hessheimer AJ, Maathuis MH, *et al.* Hypothermic oxygenated machine perfusion in porcine donation after circulatory determination of death liver transplant. Transplantation 2012; 94(1): 22-9.
[http://dx.doi.org/10.1097/TP.0b013e31825774d7] [PMID: 22691959]

[12]   Shigeta T, Matsuno N, Obara H, *et al.* Functional recovery of donation after cardiac death liver graft by continuous machine perfusion preservation in pigs. Transplant Proc 2012; 44(4): 946-7.
[http://dx.doi.org/10.1016/j.transproceed.2012.01.078] [PMID: 22564592]

[13]   Schlegel A, Graf R, Clavien PA, Dutkowski P. Hypothermic oxygenated perfusion (HOPE) protects from biliary injury in a rodent model of DCD liver transplantation. J Hepatol 2013; 59(5): 984-91.
[http://dx.doi.org/10.1016/j.jhep.2013.06.022] [PMID: 23820408]

[14]   Schlegel A, Kron P, Graf R, Clavien PA, Dutkowski P. Hypothermic Oxygenated Perfusion (HOPE) downregulates the immune response in a rat model of liver transplantation. Ann Surg 2014; 260(5): 931-7.
[http://dx.doi.org/10.1097/SLA.0000000000000941] [PMID: 25243553]

[15]   Bae C, Pichardo EM, Huang H, Henry SD, Guarrera JV. The benefits of hypothermic machine perfusion are enhanced with Vasosol and α-tocopherol in rodent donation after cardiac death livers. Transplant Proc 2014; 46(5): 1560-6.
[http://dx.doi.org/10.1016/j.transproceed.2013.12.050] [PMID: 24880463]

[16]   Op den Dries S, Sutton ME, Karimian N, *et al.* Hypothermic oxygenated machine perfusion prevents arteriolonecrosis of the peribiliary plexus in pig livers donated after circulatory death. PLoS One 2014; 9(2): e88521.
[http://dx.doi.org/10.1371/journal.pone.0088521] [PMID: 24551114]

[17]   Dutkowski P, Graf R, Clavien PA. Rescue of the cold preserved rat liver by hypothermic oxygenated machine perfusion. Am J Transplant 2006; 6(5 Pt 1): 903-12.
[http://dx.doi.org/10.1111/j.1600-6143.2006.01264.x] [PMID: 16611326]

[18]   Bessems M, Doorschodt BM, Kolkert JL, *et al.* Preservation of steatotic livers: a comparison between cold storage and machine perfusion preservation. Liver Transpl 2007; 13(4): 497-504.
[http://dx.doi.org/10.1002/lt.21039] [PMID: 17394146]

[19]   Schlegel A, de Rougemont O, Graf R, Clavien PA, Dutkowski P. Protective mechanisms of end-ischemic cold machine perfusion in DCD liver grafts. J Hepatol 2013; 58(2): 278-86.
[http://dx.doi.org/10.1016/j.jhep.2012.10.004] [PMID: 23063573]

[20]   Monbaliu D, Liu Q, Libbrecht L, *et al.* Preserving the morphology and evaluating the quality of liver grafts by hypothermic machine perfusion: a proof-of-concept study using discarded human livers. Liver Transpl 2012; 18(12): 1495-507.
[http://dx.doi.org/10.1002/lt.23550] [PMID: 22987314]

[21]   Guarrera JV. Assist devices: machine preservation of extended criteria donors. Liver Transpl 2012; 18 (Suppl. 2): S31-3.
[http://dx.doi.org/10.1002/lt.23505] [PMID: 22767437]

[22]   Vairetti M, Ferrigno A, Rizzo V, *et al.* Subnormothermic machine perfusion protects against rat liver preservation injury: a comparative evaluation with conventional cold storage. Transplant Proc 2007 2007 Jul-Aug;; 39(6): 1765-7.
[PMID: 17692606]

[23]   Vairetti M, Ferrigno A, Carlucci F, *et al.* Subnormothermic machine perfusion protects steatotic livers against preservation injury: a potential for donor pool increase? Liver Transpl 2009; 15(1): 20-9.

[http://dx.doi.org/10.1002/lt.21581] [PMID: 19109848]

[24] Okamura Y, Hata K, Tanaka H, *et al.* Impact of subnormothermic machine perfusion preservation in severely steatotic rat livers: a detailed assessment in an isolated setting. Am J Transplant 2016 Nov; Epub 2016/11/10. eng.
[PMID: 27860296]

[25] Bruinsma BG, Berendsen TA, Izamis ML, Yeh H, Yarmush ML, Uygun K. Supercooling preservation and transplantation of the rat liver. Nat Protoc 2015; 10(3): 484-94.
[http://dx.doi.org/10.1038/nprot.2015.011] [PMID: 25692985]

[26] Minor T, Efferz P, Fox M, Wohlschlaeger J, Lüer B. Controlled oxygenated rewarming of cold stored liver grafts by thermally graduated machine perfusion prior to reperfusion. Am J Transplant 2013; 13(6): 1450-60.
[http://dx.doi.org/10.1111/ajt.12235] [PMID: 23617781]

[27] Knaak JM, Spetzler VN, Goldaracena N, *et al.* Subnormothermic *ex vivo* liver perfusion reduces endothelial cell and bile duct injury after donation after cardiac death pig liver transplantation. Liver Transpl 2014; 20(11): 1296-305.
[http://dx.doi.org/10.1002/lt.23986] [PMID: 25179693]

[28] Fontes P, Lopez R, van der Plaats A, *et al.* Liver preservation with machine perfusion and a newly developed cell-free oxygen carrier solution under subnormothermic conditions. Am J Transplant 2015; 15(2): 381-94.
[http://dx.doi.org/10.1111/ajt.12991] [PMID: 25612645]

[29] Spetzler VN, Goldaracena N, Echiverri J, *et al.* Subnormothermic *ex vivo* liver perfusion is a safe alternative to cold static storage for preserving standard criteria grafts. Liver Transpl 2016; 22(1): 111-9.
[http://dx.doi.org/10.1002/lt.24340] [PMID: 26390093]

[30] Bruinsma BG, Yeh H, Ozer S, *et al.* Subnormothermic machine perfusion for *ex vivo* preservation and recovery of the human liver for transplantation. Am J Transplant 2014; 14(6): 1400-9.
[http://dx.doi.org/10.1111/ajt.12727] [PMID: 24758155]

[31] Bruinsma BG, Sridharan GV, Weeder PD, *et al.* Metabolic profiling during *ex vivo* machine perfusion of the human liver. Sci Rep 2016; 6: 22415.
[http://dx.doi.org/10.1038/srep22415] [PMID: 26935866]

[32] Whitson BA, Black SM. Organ assessment and repair centers: The future of transplantation is near. World J Transplant 2014; 4(2): 40-2.
[http://dx.doi.org/10.5500/wjt.v4.i2.40] [PMID: 25032094]

[33] Tolboom H, Izamis ML, Sharma N, *et al.* Subnormothermic machine perfusion at both 20°C and 30°C recovers ischemic rat livers for successful transplantation. J Surg Res 2012; 175(1): 149-56.
[http://dx.doi.org/10.1016/j.jss.2011.03.003] [PMID: 21550058]

[34] Hara Y, Akamatsu Y, Maida K, *et al.* A new liver graft preparation method for uncontrolled non-hear--beating donors, combining short oxygenated warm perfusion and prostaglandin E1. J Surg Res 2013; 184(2): 1134-42.
[http://dx.doi.org/10.1016/j.jss.2013.04.030] [PMID: 23688794]

[35] Nagrath D, Xu H, Tanimura Y, *et al.* Metabolic preconditioning of donor organs: defatting fatty livers by normothermic perfusion *ex vivo*. Metab Eng 2009 Jul-Sep; 11(4-5): 274-83. Epub 2009/06/07.
[PMID: 19508897] [PMCID: 2814076]

[36] Boehnert MU, Yeung JC, Bazerbachi F, *et al.* Normothermic acellular *ex vivo* liver perfusion reduces liver and bile duct injury of pig livers retrieved after cardiac death. Am J Transplant 2013; 13(6): 1441-9.
[http://dx.doi.org/10.1111/ajt.12224] [PMID: 23668775]

[37] Schön MR, Kollmar O, Wolf S, *et al.* Liver transplantation after organ preservation with

normothermic extracorporeal perfusion. Ann Surg 2001; 233(1): 114-23.
[http://dx.doi.org/10.1097/00000658-200101000-00017] [PMID: 11141233]

[38]   Reddy S, Greenwood J, Maniakin N, *et al.* Non-heart-beating donor porcine livers: the adverse effect of cooling. Liver Transpl 2005; 11(1): 35-8.
[http://dx.doi.org/10.1002/lt.20287] [PMID: 15690534]

[39]   Banan B, Xiao Z, Watson R, *et al.* Novel strategy to decrease reperfusion injuries and improve function of cold-preserved livers using normothermic *ex vivo* liver perfusion machine. Liver Transpl 2016; 22(3): 333-43.
[http://dx.doi.org/10.1002/lt.24352] [PMID: 26439190]

[40]   Brockmann J, Reddy S, Coussios C, *et al.* Normothermic perfusion: a new paradigm for organ preservation. Ann Surg 2009; 250(1): 1-6.
[http://dx.doi.org/10.1097/SLA.0b013e3181a63c10] [PMID: 19561463]

[41]   Goldaracena N, Spetzler VN, Echeverri J, *et al.* Inducing hepatitis C virus resistance after pig liver transplantation-a proof of concept of liver graft modification using warm *ex vivo* perfusion. Am J Transplant 2017; 17(4): 970-8.
[http://dx.doi.org/10.1111/ajt.14100] [PMID: 27805315]

[42]   Goldaracena N, Echeverri J, Spetzler VN, *et al.* Anti-inflammatory signaling during *ex vivo* liver perfusion improves the preservation of pig liver grafts before transplantation. Liver Transpl 2016; 22(11): 1573-83.
[http://dx.doi.org/10.1002/lt.24603] [PMID: 27556578]

[43]   op den Dries S, Karimian N, Sutton ME, *et al. Ex vivo* normothermic machine perfusion and viability testing of discarded human donor livers. Am J Transplant 2013 May; 13(5): 1327-35.
[PMID: 23463950]

[44]   Sutton ME, op den Dries S, Karimian N, *et al.* Criteria for viability assessment of discarded human donor livers during *ex vivo* normothermic machine perfusion. PLoS One 2014; 9(11): e110642.
[http://dx.doi.org/10.1371/journal.pone.0110642] [PMID: 25369327]

[45]   Reiling J, Lockwood DS, Simpson AH, *et al.* Urea production during normothermic machine perfusion: price of success? Liver Transpl 2015; 21(5): 700-3.
[http://dx.doi.org/10.1002/lt.24094] [PMID: 25690646]

[46]   Karangwa SA, Burlage LC, Adelmeijer J, *et al.* Activation of fibrinolysis, but not coagulation, during end-ischemic *ex situ* normothermic machine perfusion of human donor livers. Transplantation 2017; 101(2): e42-8.
[http://dx.doi.org/10.1097/TP.0000000000001562] [PMID: 27941437]

[47]   Ravikumar R, Jassem W, Mergental H, *et al.* Liver transplantation after *ex vivo* normothermic machine preservation: a phase 1 (first-in-man) clinical trial. Am J Transplant 2016; 16(6): 1779-87.
[http://dx.doi.org/10.1111/ajt.13708] [PMID: 26752191]

[48]   Bral M, Gala-Lopez B, Bigam D, *et al.* Preliminary single-center canadian experience of human normothermic *ex vivo* liver perfusion: results of a clinical trial. Am J Transplant 2016 Sep;
[PMID: 27639262]

[49]   Selzner M, Goldaracena N, Echeverri J, *et al.* Normothermic *ex vivo* liver perfusion using steen solution as perfusate for human liver transplantation: first North American results. Liver Transpl 2016; 22(11): 1501-8.
[http://dx.doi.org/10.1002/lt.24499] [PMID: 27339754]

[50]   Perera T, Mergental H, Stephenson B, *et al.* First human liver transplantation using a marginal allograft resuscitated by normothermic machine perfusion. Liver Transpl 2016; 22(1): 120-4.
[http://dx.doi.org/10.1002/lt.24369] [PMID: 26566737]

[51]   Watson CJ, Randle LV, Kosmoliaptsis V, Gibbs P, Allison M, Butler AJ. 26-hour storage of a declined liver before successful transplantation using *ex vivo* normothermic perfusion. Ann Surg 2017;

265(1): e1-2.
[http://dx.doi.org/10.1097/SLA.0000000000001834] [PMID: 27295096]

[52]   Mergental H, Perera MT, Laing RW, *et al.* Transplantation of declined liver allografts following normothermic *ex situ* evaluation. Am J Transplant 2016; 16(11): 3235-45.
[http://dx.doi.org/10.1111/ajt.13875] [PMID: 27192971]

[53]   Watson CJ, Kosmoliaptsis V, Randle LV, *et al.* Preimplant normothermic liver perfusion of a suboptimal liver donated after circulatory death. Am J Transplant 2016; 16(1): 353-7.
[http://dx.doi.org/10.1111/ajt.13448] [PMID: 26393945]

[54]   Black SM, Whitson BA, Velayutham M. EPR spectroscopy as a predictive tool for the assessment of marginal donor livers perfused on a normothermic *ex vivo* perfusion circuit. Med Hypotheses 2014; 82(5): 627-30.
[http://dx.doi.org/10.1016/j.mehy.2014.02.025] [PMID: 24629357]

[55]   Averkiou M, Keravnou CP, Izamis ML, Leen E. Evaluation of perfusion quantification methods with ultrasound contrast agents in a machine-perfused pig liver. Ultraschall Med 2016 May;
[PMID: 27139375]

[56]   Shaver CM, Ware LB. Primary graft dysfunction: pathophysiology to guide new preventive therapies. Expert Rev Respir Med 2017; 11(2): 119-28.
[http://dx.doi.org/10.1080/17476348.2017.1280398] [PMID: 28074663]

[57]   Martens A, Van Raemdonck DE, Smits J, *et al.* A retrospective database analysis to evaluate the potential of *ex vivo* lung perfusion to recruit declined lung donors. Transpl Int 2017 May;
[PMID: 28556538]

[58]   Cypel M, Yeung JC, Liu M, *et al.* Normothermic *ex vivo* lung perfusion in clinical lung transplantation. N Engl J Med 2011; 364(15): 1431-40.
[http://dx.doi.org/10.1056/NEJMoa1014597] [PMID: 21488765]

[59]   Spratt JR, Mattison LM, Iaizzo PA, *et al.* An experimental study of the recovery of injured porcine lungs with prolonged normothermic cellular *ex vivo* lung perfusion following donation after circulatory death. Transpl Int 2017 May; Epub 2017/05/11.
[PMID: 28493634]

[60]   Charles EJ, Mehaffey JH, Sharma AK, *et al.* Lungs donated after circulatory death and prolonged warm ischemia are transplanted successfully after enhanced *ex vivo* lung perfusion using adenosine A2B receptor antagonism. J Thorac Cardiovasc Surg 2017 Apr; Epub 2017/04/12.
[PMID: 28483262]

[61]   Machuca TN, Cypel M, Bonato R, *et al.* Safety and efficacy of *ex vivo* donor lung adenoviral IL-10 gene therapy in a large animal lung transplant survival model. Hum Gene Ther 2017 Jan; Epub 2017/01/04.
[PMID: 28052693]

[62]   Nakajima D, Liu M, Ohsumi A, *et al.* Lung Lavage and surfactant replacement during *ex vivo* lung perfusion for treatment of gastric acid aspiration-induced donor lung injury. J Heart Lung Transplant 2017; 36(5): 577-85.
[http://dx.doi.org/10.1016/j.healun.2016.11.010] [PMID: 28041954]

[63]   Mehaffey JH, Charles EJ, Sharma AK, *et al. Ex vivo* lung perfusion rehabilitates sepsis-induced lung injury. Ann Thorac Surg 2017 Apr; Epub 2017/04/20.
[PMID: 28434548]

[64]   Martens A, Ordies S, Vanaudenaerde BM, *et al.* Immunoregulatory effects of multipotent adult progenitor cells in a porcine *ex vivo* lung perfusion model. Stem Cell Res Ther 2017; 8(1): 159.
[http://dx.doi.org/10.1186/s13287-017-0603-5] [PMID: 28676074]

[65]   Martens A, Boada M, Vanaudenaerde BM, *et al.* Steroids can reduce warm ischemic reperfusion injury in a porcine donation after circulatory death model with *ex vivo* lung perfusion evaluation.

Transpl Int 2016; 29(11): 1237-46.
[http://dx.doi.org/10.1111/tri.12823] [PMID: 27514498]

[66]   Bassani GA, Lonati C, Brambilla D, Rapido F, Valenza F, Gatti S. *Ex vivo* lung perfusion in the rat: detailed procedure and videos. PLoS One 2016; 11(12): e0167898.
[http://dx.doi.org/10.1371/journal.pone.0167898] [PMID: 27936178]

[67]   Noda K, Tane S, Haam SJ, *et al.* Optimal *ex vivo* lung perfusion techniques with oxygenated perfusate. J Heart Lung Transplant 2017; 36(4): 466-74.
[http://dx.doi.org/10.1016/j.healun.2016.10.014] [PMID: 27914896]

[68]   Noda K, Tane S, Haam SJ, *et al.* Targeting circulating leukocytes and pyroptosis during *ex vivo* lung perfusion improves lung preservation. Transplantation 2017 Apr; Epub 2017/04/27.
[PMID: 28452921]

[69]   Luc JG, Aboelnazar NS, Himmat S, *et al.* A leukocyte filter does not provide further benefit during *ex vivo* lung perfusion. ASAIO J 2017 Feb; Epub 2017/02/20.
[PMID: 28234641]

[70]   Francioli C, Wang X, Parapanov R, *et al.* Pyrrolidine dithiocarbamate administered during *ex vivo* lung perfusion promotes rehabilitation of injured donor rat lungs obtained after prolonged warm ischemia. PLoS One 2017; 12(3): e0173916.
[http://dx.doi.org/10.1371/journal.pone.0173916] [PMID: 28323904]

[71]   Wang X, Wang Y, Parapanov R, *et al.* Pharmacological reconditioning of marginal donor rat lungs using inhibitors of peroxynitrite and poly (ADP-ribose) polymerase during *ex vivo* lung perfusion. Transplantation 2016; 100(7): 1465-73.
[http://dx.doi.org/10.1097/TP.0000000000001183] [PMID: 27331361]

[72]   Fisher A, Andreasson A, Chrysos A, *et al.* An observational study of Donor *ex vivo* lung perfusion in UK lung transplantation: DEVELOP-UK. Health Technol Assess 2016; 20(85): 1-276.
[http://dx.doi.org/10.3310/hta20850] [PMID: 27897967]

[73]   Yeung JC, Krueger T, Yasufuku K, *et al.* Outcomes after transplantation of lungs preserved for more than 12 h: a retrospective study. Lancet Respir Med 2017; 5(2): 119-24.
[http://dx.doi.org/10.1016/S2213-2600(16)30323-X] [PMID: 27866861]

[74]   Wallinder A, Riise GC, Ricksten SE, Silverborn M, Dellgren G. Transplantation after *ex vivo* lung perfusion: A midterm follow-up. J Heart Lung Transplant 2016; 35(11): 1303-10.
[http://dx.doi.org/10.1016/j.healun.2016.05.021] [PMID: 27381674]

[75]   Shafaghi S, Mortaz E, Abbasi Dezfuli A, *et al.* Normothermic *ex vivo* lung perfusion in brain-dead donors reduces inflammatory cytokines and toll-like receptor expression. Iran J Allergy Asthma Immunol 2016; 15(5): 340-54.
[PMID: 27917620]

[76]   Nakajima D, Cypel M, Bonato R, *et al.* Ex vivo perfusion treatment of infection in human donor lungs. Am J Transplant 2016; 16(4): 1229-37.
[http://dx.doi.org/10.1111/ajt.13562] [PMID: 26730551]

[77]   Hashimoto K, Cypel M, Juvet S, *et al.* Higher M30 and high mobility group box 1 protein levels in *ex vivo* lung perfusate are associated with primary graft dysfunction after human lung transplantation. J Heart Lung Transplant 2017 Jun; Epub 2017/06/21.
[PMID: 28689646]

[78]   Maignan M, Gennai S, Debaty G, *et al.* Exhaled carbon monoxide is correlated with ischemia reperfusion injuries during *ex vivo* lung perfusion in pigs. J Breath Res 2017 Jun; Epub 2017/06/20.
[PMID: 28631618]

[79]   Andreasson ASI, Borthwick LA, Gillespie C, *et al.* The role of interleukin-1β as a predictive biomarker and potential therapeutic target during clinical *ex vivo* lung perfusion. J Heart Lung Transplant 2017 May; Epub 2017/05/12.

[PMID: 28551353]

[80]   Sage E, De Wolf J, Puyo P, *et al.* Real-time computed tomography highlights pulmonary parenchymal evolution during *ex vivo* lung reconditioning. Ann Thorac Surg 2017; 103(6): e535-7.
[http://dx.doi.org/10.1016/j.athoracsur.2016.12.029] [PMID: 28528061]

[81]   Slama A, Schillab L, Barta M, *et al.* Standard donor lung procurement with normothermic *ex vivo* lung perfusion: A prospective randomized clinical trial. J Heart Lung Transplant 2017 Feb; Epub 2017/02/20.
[PMID: 28314503]

[82]   Cypel M, Yeung JC, Machuca T, *et al.* Experience with the first 50 *ex vivo* lung perfusions in clinical transplantation. J Thorac Cardiovasc Surg 2012; 144(5): 1200-6.
[http://dx.doi.org/10.1016/j.jtcvs.2012.08.009] [PMID: 22944089]

[83]   Tikkanen JM, Cypel M, Machuca TN, *et al.* Functional outcomes and quality of life after normothermic *ex vivo* lung perfusion lung transplantation. J Heart Lung Transplant 2015; 34(4): 547-56.
[http://dx.doi.org/10.1016/j.healun.2014.09.044] [PMID: 25476845]

[84]   Boffini M, Ricci D, Bonato R, *et al.* Incidence and severity of primary graft dysfunction after lung transplantation using rejected grafts reconditioned with *ex vivo* lung perfusion. Eur J Cardiothorac Surg 2014; 46(5): 789-93.
[http://dx.doi.org/10.1093/ejcts/ezu239] [PMID: 25061216]

[85]   Sage E, Mussot S, Trebbia G, *et al.* Foch Lung Transplant Group. Lung transplantation from initially rejected donors after *ex vivo* lung reconditioning: the French experience. Eur J Cardiothorac Surg 2014; 46(5): 794-9.
[http://dx.doi.org/10.1093/ejcts/ezu245] [PMID: 25061219]

[86]   Machuca TN, Mercier O, Collaud S, *et al.* Lung transplantation with donation after circulatory determination of death donors and the impact of *ex vivo* lung perfusion. Am J Transplant 2015; 15(4): 993-1002.
[http://dx.doi.org/10.1111/ajt.13124] [PMID: 25772069]

[87]   Reeb J, Cypel M. *Ex vivo* lung perfusion. Clin Transplant 2016; 30(3): 183-94.
[http://dx.doi.org/10.1111/ctr.12680] [PMID: 26700566]

[88]   Henkenberens C, Zinne N, Biancosino C, *et al.* A new era of thoracic oncology? *ex vivo* stereotactic ablative radiosurgery within *ex vivo* lung treatment system as a hybrid therapy for unresectable locally advanced pulmonary malignancies. Med Hypotheses 2016; 92: 31-4.
[http://dx.doi.org/10.1016/j.mehy.2016.04.029] [PMID: 27241251]

[89]   Krüger M, Zinne N, Biancosino C, *et al.* Porcine pulmonary auto-transplantation for *ex vivo* therapy as a model for new treatment strategies. Interact Cardiovasc Thorac Surg 2016; 23(3): 358-66.
[http://dx.doi.org/10.1093/icvts/ivw160] [PMID: 27230537]

[90]   Cypel M, Keshavjee S. Novel technologies for isolated lung perfusion: beyond lung transplant. Thorac Surg Clin 2016; 26(2): 139-45.
[http://dx.doi.org/10.1016/j.thorsurg.2015.12.002] [PMID: 27112253]

CHAPTER 15

The Future of Organ Donation and Transplantation: 2018 and Beyond

Robert S.D. Higgins[*]

Johns Hopkins University School of Medicine, Baltimore, MD, USA

Organ donation after brain death, donation after cardiac death, and living donation are the cornerstones of solid organ and islet cell transplantation in a transplant field dependent upon a precious supply of viable, high quality organs, which if well managed, can save thousands of lives every day. The future will bring increased utilization of organs from donors not previously viewed as suitable due to age and other factors (*i.e.* Hepatitis C and HIV). As such, selecting and managing potential donors is more important now than ever. *Ex vivo* organ perfusion support, partial organ transplants and mechanical/artificial organs will fill the void left by the inadequate supply of viable organs.

Logistical considerations reviewed in this text and other articles by Engelsby and Marion [1] highlight the importance of risks associated with procurement travel and the safety precautions necessary for transplant and organ procurement professionals to avoid catastrophic occurrences. Organ quality and preservation must be balanced with these time-sensitive logistics to avoid organ waste, or managed with established and evolving supportive strategies, such as mechanical pump or *ex vivo* preservation.

The Organ Procurement and Transplant Network (OPTN) established in 2000 through its Final Rule, stipulates that "allocation policies must among other factors be based on sound medical judgement, seek to achieve the best use of donated organs, and shall not be based on the candidates' place of residence or place of listing except to the extent needed to satisfy other regulatory requirements [2].

Ongoing policy discussions and recent legal challenges to meet these stipulations have made significant effort to enhance broader sharing of donated organs in the liver, heart and lung allocation policies authored by the United Network For Organ Sharing (UNOS), the elected group of transplant professionals from around

---

[*] **Corresponding author Robert S.D. Higgins:** Johns Hopkins University School of Medicine, Baltimore, MD, USA; Tel: 443-287-3497; Fax: 443-769-1273; Email: robert.higgins@jhmi.edu

the country who serve on the OPTN Board of Directors. In spite of efforts to strike a balance of equity in access, improve outcomes and limit the impact on travel and procurement logistics, the OPTN/UNOS Board of Directors has instructed all organ-specific committees to identify allocation equity metrics appropriate to their organ types. The OPTN recognizes that there are not enough organs for patients in need of lifesaving transplants and invests in increasing the number of transplants each year by increasing donation, reducing organ discards, and improving Organ Procurement Organization performance.

The development of recipient disease severity scoring systems in adult and pediatric patients, Model for End-Stage Liver Disease (MELD) or if less than 12 years old, Pediatric End Stage Liver Disease , (PELD) and the Lung Allocation Score (LAS) have helped to predict the risk of 3-month mortality without access to heart, liver or lung transplant. However, the existing geographic disparities in allocation of organs for transplantation continue to be unacceptably high. The Thoracic Organ Transplantation Committee recently proposed modifications to better stratify the most medically urgent heart transplant candidates reflecting the use of mechanical circulatory support devices including veno-arterial extracorporeal membrane oxygenation and other temporary devices.

In spite of these efforts, a family in New York has recently sued the Secretary of HHS in federal court based on disparities in access in the lung allocation system. In response, the HRSA administrator charged the OPTN/UNOS board with determining whether the lung allocation policy was consistent with the principles of allocation in accordance with the Final Rule. In response to the HRSA directive, because lung distribution was based on the Donor Service Area (DSA) regardless of medical urgency, the OPTN/UNOS Board took the unprecedented action of changing lung allocation policy and reprogramming allocation in less than 7 days. Consonant with that approach, the following week, the UNOS board approved the liver allocation sharing plan that was developed through consensus over a long and difficult period.

As stewards of these precious life-saving organs, transplant professionals using this text including nurses, trainees, residents , fellows and faculty will be well equipped to optimize the identification, preservation, procurement and implantation of viable, high quality organs and cells for transplantation. We also expect that with advances in cellular and *ex vivo* preservation techniques as well as better consensus-driven, time-sensitive allocation policy improvements focusing on access and equity for those in greatest need we will continue to save lives.

CONSENT FOR PUBLICATION

Not applicable.

CONFLICT OF INTEREST

The author declares no conflict of interest, financial or otherwise.

ACKNOWLEDGEMENTS

Declared none.

REFERENCES

[1]   42 C.F.R 121.8, US department of health & human services (http://www.hhs.gov/).

[2]   Engesbe M. Merion, R. The riskiest job in medicine-transplant surgeons and organ procurement travel. Am J Transplant 2009; 2406-15.
       [http://dx.doi.org/10.1111/j.1600-6143.2009.02774.x]

SUBJECT INDEX

A

Abdomen, donor's 128, 129, 131
Abdominal cavity 103, 104, 109, 113, 119
ABO 91, 92
  compatibility 91, 92
  -compatible donors 92
  -identical donors 92
Absolute contraindications 53, 54, 92, 117,
    161
  for organ donation 161
ACIN system 20, 21
Allocation 13, 14, 152
  for adult donors 13, 14
  systems, government-led deceased donor
    152
AOPO confirmation information network
    (ACIN) 20
Apnea test 26, 28, 29, 33, 34, 35, 36, 39
Aspiration 56, 94, 177
  gastric acid 177
Assessment of kidney donor candidates 138
Association of organ procurement
    organizations (AOPO) 7, 164

B

Biliary complications 70, 72, 128, 151, 154,
    155, 169, 174
Biliary 131, 149, 150
  radicles 149, 150
  tree 131
Body mass index (BMI) 82, 117, 126, 137,
    138, 139, 160, 162, 163
Body surface area (BSA) 82, 162, 163
Brain death 24, 26, 27, 29, 36, 80, 94
  determination 24, 80
  evaluations 26, 94
  examination 26, 27, 29, 36

Brainstem death 39, 53
Brain tumor, primary 161

Bronchiolitis obliterans syndrome (BOS) 92,
    178
Bronchoalveolar lavage 179
Bronchoscopy 11, 56, 93, 95
BSA, included donor 163

C

Calculated panel reactive antibody (CPRA)
    16, 17, 18, 19
Cannulas, aortic 108, 109, 119
Cardiac 11, 25, 67, 81, 99, 116, 117, 161, 162,
    189
  arrest 25, 162
  death 25, 99, 116, 117, 161, 189
  enzymes 11, 81
  grafts 67
Cardiothoracic surgeries 118
Carrell patch of aorta 112
Catecholamine surge 56
Catell-Braash maneuver 104, 105
Caucasian donors 142
CDC high risk donors 45
Central venous pressure (CVP) 11, 55, 83
Cessation, irreversible 25
Cholangiogram 129, 130, 131, 133, 134
Cholecystectomy 107, 129, 131, 134
Code of federal regulations (CFR) 5
Coercion, emotional donor 137
Cold ischemia times 71, 122, 161, 162, 179
Common bile duct (CBD) 106, 107, 114, 118,
    121
Computed tomography (CT) 37, 126, 127, 179
  angiography (CTA) 37
Coronary angiogram 81
Crystal city guidelines 81, 83

D

Deceased donor 10, 135, 147
  organ procurement 10
  split liver procurement 147

.

www.ingramcontent.com/pod-product-compliance
Lightning Source LLC
Chambersburg PA
CBHW050841220326
41598CB00006B/429